A Time
to be Born,

A Time
to Die

Rasa Gustaitis is the author of
Turning On and
Wholly Round.

A Time to be Born,

A Time to Die

CONFLICTS and ETHICS in an Intensive Care Nursery

Rasa Gustaitis
and
Ernlé W. D. Young

Reading, Massachusetts · Menlo Park, California
Don Mills, Ontario · Wokingham, England · Amsterdam
Sydney · Singapore · Tokyo · Madrid · Bogotá
Santiago · San Juan

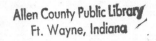
Page 187: Reprinted by permission from the *New England Journal of Medicine* 309 (1983): excerpt from "Handicapped Children: Baby Doe and Uncle Sam" by Marcia Angell, p. 660.
Page 242: Reprinted by permission from the *New England Journal of Medicine* 309 (1983): excerpt from "Parents and Handicapped Infants," by Helen Harrison, pp. 664–5.

Library of Congress Cataloging-in-Publication Data

Gustaitis, Rasa.
  A time to be born, a time to die.

  Includes index.
  1. Neonatal intensive care—Economic aspects.
2. Neonatal intensive care—Moral and ethical
aspects. 3. Neonatal intensive care—Decision making.
I. Young, Ernlé W. D. II. Title.
RJ253.5.G87 1986   362.1′9892′01   85-26804
ISBN 0–201–11555–7

Cover design by Marge Anderson
Text design by Kenneth J. Wilson
Set in 10 point Bookman Light ITC by Compset, Inc., Beverly, MA

ABCDEFGHIJ-DO-89876

CONTENTS

7099231

To every thing there is a season, and a time to every purpose
under the heaven;
A time to be born, and a time to die; a time to plant, and a
time to pluck up that which is planted;
A time to kill, and a time to heal; a time to break down, and a
time to build up;
A time to weep, and a time to laugh; a time to mourn and a
time to dance;
A time to cast away stones, and a time to gather stones
together; a time to embrace, and a time to refrain from
embracing;
A time to get, and a time to lose; a time to keep, and a time to
cast away;
A time to rend, and a time to sew; a time to keep silence, and
a time to speak;
A time to love, and a time to hate; a time of war, and a time of
peace.

—Ecclesiastes 3:1–8

ACKNOWLEDGMENTS

This book exists because physicians, nurses, social service staff, and others at the Stanford University Medical Center accepted into their midst and allowed an outsider to watch and listen, even during tense and difficult moments, and because many of the staff were willing to share their experiences, thoughts, hopes, and anxieties about the work in which they were engaged.

Very special thanks are due to Dr. Ronald L. Ariagno, who opened the door to this research and spent many hours answering questions and reviewing the manuscript, to ensure that medical and other facts were correctly presented. Any errors are ours.

Dr. Philip Sunshine, director of nurseries, and associate directors Dr. David Stevenson and Dr. William Benitz were always available to clarify and discuss fine points and they were most generous with their time. The same held true for the neonatology fellows, Drs. Philip James, Michael Trautman, and Terrence J. Sweeney. Special thanks to Dr. William L. Salomon for his editorial help.

Many other physicians contributed; they include Peter Gorski, Gary E. Hartman, David Kasting, Karen Kral, Cynthia Meyers-Seifer, William Oh, Mark Ovadia, Niels C. R. Raïha, Martha Reitman, Rosebeth Rosen, Lynn Scannell, Jeffrey Schneider, Stephen J. Shochat, and Craig Wilson. Dr. Alison Kallman was especially helpful in research on medical costs. Dr. Dwayne Reed was an important catalyst for this project in the mid-1970s when, while chief of the epidemiology branch at the National Institute of Child Health and Human Development, he pointed out that premature infants who survived with the help of intensive care had a much higher incidence of childhood illness than infants in general.

No one attempted to censor any portion of this text, even when he or she disagreed with the authors' interpretation or point of view, or when something seemed to reflect negatively on them, or the medical center. For this we acknowledge our highest respect and regard. We recognize that in the current political and social climate, their open attitude involved taking risks.

Acknowledgments

The social support staff and nurses were patient, friendly, and frank. Our many thanks go to Kathy Petersen for indispensable and varied help on numerous occasions, to Charlene Canger and Ken Pinhero for sharing their tiny office space and responding obligingly to our many requests for assistance. Our thanks also to Rose Grobstein, Maria Najleti, Elizabeth Plata-Wilson; to nurses Denise Carter, Sandy Chapman, Ilene Craft, Cathy Garaventa, Susan Hammel, Gayle Hand, Judy Kandel, Jeri Lange, Barbara Magee, Caroline Miyagishima, Dian Ruder, Pat Scheid, Beverly Squaglia, Cathy Van Buren, Nancy Vierhaus, Vicki Welsh, Lilly Yoshida, and others on the nursing staff; to respiratory therapists Darlene Allen and Dan Proud; to public health nurses Cheryl Barton, Marie Heid, Sandy Standing, and Loretta Young; and to physical therapist Lorraine McCleary. We are indebted to physical therapist Cathy Adachi for much of the information in Chapter Nine, to other therapists and teachers at the George Miller Center. Clifford R. Barnett, professor of anthropology, helped with a cross-cultural bibliography.

The contributions of the babies' parents are gratefully acknowledged. Some parents consented to talk about the most poignant experiences in their lives, in the hope of helping others, even though the interviews revived their pain.

Frank Doran and Robert Nadeau provided guidance in keeping us on course. Peter and Joanne Carey offered warm overnight hospitality in their home; they also aided in our struggle to learn to use a computer. Curt Philips walked a panicked author through some computer crises. Mery Clausen, Linda Judd, and Helen Wada kindly relayed messages and information. Our families were forbearing.

Robert Lavelle is the editor writers hope to find. His suggestions were consistently on the mark. He understood what we were reaching for and helped us to get there.

PREFACE

In July 1984, an article was published in *Pediatrics*, the leading journal in the field, on a subject that some readers considered unseemly or even crude. A cost-benefit analysis of intensive care for very small and premature newborns, it indirectly posed the question, Does it make sense to try to save babies born so early that their survival requires months of aggressive life support?[1]

This question greatly concerned health professionals familiar with recent developments in high-risk nurseries. But it was rarely faced full-on in the literature, particularly not in economic terms. The authors of this article offered data that they hoped might prove useful in discussions that were sure to become more heated as medical cost-cutting continued.

Using the records of 247 infants who weighed between 500 and 999 grams at birth and were admitted to Women and Infants Hospital of Rhode Island between January 1977 and December 1981, Drs. Donna-Jean B. Walker, Allan Feldman, Betty R. Vohr, and William Oh balanced estimated costs of the care they received versus their estimated lifetime earnings.

More than two-thirds (68 percent) of these infants died shortly after birth. The survivors were divided into groups by birth weight, and costs were calculated for their lifetime needs, including newborn intensive care, education, physical therapy, custodial care, and therapy for the handicapped. The total estimated costs were balanced against estimated earning capacities. The conclusion: from the standpoint of the cost-benefit analysis used in the study, newborn intensive care may not be justifiable for infants weighing less than 900 grams—just under two pounds—at birth.

Three months after the study was published, coauthor Oh presented some of its data to the World Symposium of Perinatal Medicine, which brought more than five hundred of his colleagues to the Marriott Hotel near the White House. He pointed out that more than 50 percent of infants born weighing more than 900 grams survived, and that 85 percent of those who lived developed

normally. Below that birth weight, society's investment of resources was not likely to yield a net benefit in economic terms.
And the smaller and more premature the survivors, the greater
their chances of serious handicap and lifelong dependency.

By presenting this analysis, Dr. Oh had opened the door for the
most difficult and controversial question in medicine today: At
what point does aggressive life saving cease to be beneficial and
begin to be harmful? Clearly, the question is one of ethics as well
as economics. The economic framework is simply one way to look
at data that involves much pain and suffering. Dr. Oh had, indirectly, broached a subject that was engendering increasing
concern.

Nobody seized the opportunity to engage in a wider discussion.
The subject is so explosive that physicians tend to avoid talking
about it, except in small groups. After answering a few desultory
questions about methodology and statistics, Dr. Oh stepped
down from the podium, to be succeeded by a series of specialists
who spoke of new interventions into labor and delivery, management of premature infants, and treatment of complicated pregnancies. Philosophical considerations were not explored—except
during coffee breaks and outside the formal sessions—at this six-
day conference.

Everywhere, however, conscientious obstetricians, pediatricians, parents, legislators, and others worry about the moral dilemmas that shadow medical progress. In the 1950s, little could
be done for a baby born weighing three pounds, even in the most
modern medical centers. The infant was usually put into an incubator, given extra oxygen, fed, and watched. Some survived;
most did not. Now a three-pounder is a very large baby in an intensive care nursery and infants scarcely heavier than a pound—
who would have become miscarriages not long ago—are kept alive
with the help of costly and elaborate technology. Nobody knows
what kinds of adults they will grow up to be. Some will have serious disabilities.

How should the principle of preserving life be weighed against
the medical community's commitment to do no harm and to alleviate suffering? This is the most basic issue in medicine today.
It needs to be more widely discussed, for everyone's benefit.

Like the article by Dr. Walker and her colleagues, this book is
one more effort to consider this issue as it arises at life's threshold. More than to evaluate or prescribe, we seek to show the real-

ities of newborns, families, and caregivers who are at the center of controversies in the intensive care nursery. We also sketch some guidelines that may aid in sorting out the ethics of decision making on yet-to-be-charted terrain.

Intensive care for infants at the threshold of viability is established as a national choice. Readers of this book may legitimately begin to wonder, as we do, whether intensive care is always the wisest choice. One thing is certain: national preferences are shaped and can be changed by public opinion. To the extent that this book seeks to inform public opinion in one important area, we hope it will become an instrument for changing public policy.

We invite you to take an intimate look at the leading edge of neonatology, a field that, in itself, represents a leading edge in American medicine. We focus on one of the most advanced medical facilities, the Stanford University Medical Center Intensive Care Nursery (ICN), where the staff is dedicated and highly competent, equipment is state-of-the- art, and the patient population is diverse and representative.

This book grew from a confluence of our long interest in the value questions raised by advances in medical technologies that affect the newborn and the unborn. Ernlé Young had been facing these questions in the course of his work as chaplain and ethicist at the medical center. Rasa Gustaitis had been reporting on them for Pacific News Service. We met in the autumn of 1983, when Gustaitis, then a professional journalism fellow at Stanford University, attended a medical ethics seminar taught by Young.

With the gracious permission of Dr. Ronald L. Ariagno, associate director of nurseries at Stanford, Gustaitis began to attend doctors' rounds in the ICN. By spring 1984, the book project had evolved. Young agreed to provide a theological and philosophical framework for examination of the issues raised by Gustaitis' research.

During the eighteen months that ended in the summer of 1985, Gustaitis watched, listened, asked questions of staff, engaged in conversations, and conducted formal interviews in and around the ICN. She repeatedly visited parents at home, usually before and after infants were discharged from the hospital. She talked with community health professionals and scholars. The pages that follow reflect what she learned. Most of the patients and families, and a few of the doctors, nurses, and other staff members, have been given pseudonyms to protect their privacy.

By examining one of the best ICNs in the world, undistracted by deficiencies that might be specific to less advanced institutions, we should be able to discover fundamental issues. As the story unfolds, many will arise. We hope to stimulate reflection on what happens in intensive care nurseries and, beyond them, in society at large.

Part One

The

Intensive Care

Nursery

CHAPTER ONE

First Questions:

A Matter of Choice

When Mariel Lew was four months pregnant, she dreamed she was terribly thirsty. Her throat was parched. Searching for water she came upon a woman who offered her a drink from a long-handled dipper. Mariel drank and was returning the dipper when she saw a large worm inside it. In horror, her hand went to her mouth. She touched something long, thin, and alien. It was not a worm, however; it was the tail of a mouse. She pulled, but it would not come out. She pulled desperately, with all her power, but the creature worked its way down into her throat, and she could not dislodge it. She was choking.

When she woke, her jaws hurt from the struggle. She marked the date of the dream in her diary, sensing that it was somehow important, but then tried to forget it. She did not tell her husband about it, lest by recognizing it she give it power. Pregnant women have all kinds of vivid dreams, she told herself. But the dream stayed with her, and when she found a dead mouse under her refrigerator one evening, she was terrified by what she thought was another dark portent.

Mariel prayed for the coming child, her second. Her first son had been born deaf. She prayed that this baby would arrive healthy and sound, and she concentrated on helping her husband who, with members of both their families, was in the process of acquiring a small retail sales business. Its success was essential, for they had bought a pleasant small house in one of the new subdivisions that had sprung up throughout the Santa Clara Valley, which had been known for its orchards before becoming world famous as the Silicon Valley, heartland of the fast-changing electronics industry. The Lews had come from Southeast Asia. Many of their neighbors were also immigrants, from Latin America, Pacific island nations, India, the Arab world, and elsewhere—recent settlers in California, where the Horatio Alger myth was still valid for those who were bold, skilled, hard-working, and lucky entrepreneurs. The Lews' detached house, with its patch of lawn, was at the end of a cul-de-sac. From the front door, mountains were visible. A handsome new school, surrounded by green playing fields, was only a short walk away. Here children could grow up safely and prepare to meet the demands of the future.

Chris Lew was born with tracheal stenosis, a rare condition that is almost invariably fatal. His windpipe was too narrow to allow him to breathe adequately. The physicians who delivered him at a nearby hospital believed he would surely expire, knew no way to help, and called the experts at the Stanford University Medical Center for a second opinion.

Surgeons at Stanford decided to try tracheoplasty—widening the trachea through plastic surgery, using cartilage from elsewhere in the body—a risky procedure that, as far as they knew, had never been performed on a newborn. They knew that the operation had been attempted on some older children, but without encouraging results. It was a long shot, but they thought it was worth a try with this baby, especially since he seemed to be normal except for this particular defect. Chris was taken to Stanford.

After examining the baby, the surgeons told the parents they had very little choice. Either the baby would recover and be relatively normal or he would not survive. The Lews signed consent forms. The complex operation took about eight hours. So the water of hope was offered to Mariel Lew. As in her dream, she soon saw the horror that accompanied it.

Three weeks after his birth, Chris was in the intensive care nursery (ICN), sprawled on his back, his arms and legs limp, immobile under warming lamps. His skin was bluish; there was a great deal of surgical tape on his chest and torso. He was hooked to a respirator, an intravenous (IV) line, and to cardiorespiratory monitors. He looked dead. Only his chest moved. He had been paralyzed with Pavulon—pancuronium—a drug that completely relaxes the muscles. Above his head a sign called attention to the endotracheal (ET) tube through which he was being ventilated: "Guard ET tube carefully. Do not retape. Do not reposition."

Chris was powerless to move or cry, but he continued to hear, see, and feel. Speculation on what he and other babies on Pavulon experience is a matter of controversy among physicians.

Surgeons at Stanford, and in many American hospitals, generally do not prescribe pain-relieving drugs for infants so paralyzed after operations because they believe that intravenously administered sedatives carry the risk of serious side effects. They explain that they have seen babies who were medicated with narcotics, after straightforward operations such as hernia repair, develop respiratory arrest and die or suffer severe brain damage. Neonatologists counter by pointing out that the surgeons cite anecdotal evidence, not studies, to support their belief. They see far less risk of side effects and prescribe pain relievers routinely.

The magnitude of the risk is not known because it has not been well documented; nor has the effect of not giving pain relievers to infants. So physicians' stands on this issue may depend on the value they place on their goal of a successful surgical outcome, relative to their concern for alleviating pain caused by treatment.

What allows the surgeons to be at ease with this policy is their belief that infants feel pain to a far lesser degree than older persons do. This is another point of disagreement between them and neonatologists, and obstetricians and anesthesiologists. Asked how they know what an infant who can neither move nor cry feels, the surgeons reply that signals from the autonomic nervous system translate into readings of blood pressure, heart rate, and oxygen diffusion. But this is a volatile issue about which it is hard to be objective and impossible to be unemotional. The Stanford surgeons believe they take the safe rather than what appears to be the humane route.

Nurses, who are their closest and most persistent observers, perceive that the babies under Pavulon suffer. Many nurses have approached the surgeons to try to persuade them of their view, but they have not succeeded. All involved in this particular controversy hope that the infants will forget whatever they feel.

The prolonged use of Pavulon can cause many problems. The drug slows blood flow and leads to edema: the capillaries leak; the body retains fluids and swells. Muscles may contract and become resistant to stretching, or they may atrophy. Some researchers have warned that seizures may go undetected. Pavulon is prescribed to conserve infants' energies, to stabilize them, to permit mechanical ventilation without patient resistance, and to keep the infant from dislodging stitches, needles, or equipment. It is one of the many useful but risky ICN interventions.

"They won't know for a while if the operation was successful," said Chris's nurse. "He's been Pavulonized since day one. After we take him off, it will be a while before we get the diaphragm moving. That's when they can extubate [remove the endotracheal tube] and find out if it worked."

Chris was paralyzed for a month. Then he had a series of setbacks that prolonged his time on the respirator. He developed a bacterial infection, then a viral infection. Later, a new problem, hydrocephalus—an abnormal buildup of fluids in the brain's ventricles—was identified. This may have been a congenital condition or the result of an infection that impeded normal circulation and absorption of cerebrospinal fluids. When his ventilator support was withdrawn, the surgeons were pleased to find that their operation had been a success: what had been the narrowest part of his windpipe, below the vocal cords, had been widened. But now the upper part was constricted, probably as an adverse effect of the intubation. In addition, a computerized axial tomography (CAT) scan showed neurological damage. Whether that was congenital or had been caused by illness or treatment could not then be determined. Because of the baby's condition, no electroencephalogram (EEG) had been taken before surgery. But it was apparent that Chris would be impaired—to what degree would remain unclear—and possibly suffer from cerebral palsy (CP) and mental retardation. He had begun to show spastic tremors.

When Mariel first saw her paralyzed baby son, she was certain that he was dead. The doctors explained that his condition was a temporary and necessary result of his therapy. She smiled politely at the doctors and nurses and thanked them for their efforts in behalf of Chris. But when she went home she cried.

Because Chris was a surgical patient, he was bypassed when the neonatologists, who were responsible for most of the other babies in the nursery, made their daily rounds. How responsibility for patients is divided in an ICN varies among institutions. In some, surgeons relinquish control of patients to the neonatologists. At Stanford, surgeons tend to retain control of infants on whom they have operated. Some medical team members were uneasy, watching this baby, but they knew about territorial rights.

The surgeons might consult with other physicians, but they had a different slant on what was in a baby's best interest. "Surgeons tend to see babies as sets of correctable parts," a nursery staff member once remarked. In Chris's case, they had corrected the targeted defect but subsequently found themselves facing a plethora of problems.

After Chris no longer needed the ventilator, he could breathe only with the help of an ET tube inserted into his nose and passed through the tight section of his upper trachea to his larynx. It was held in place by three pieces of tape. One went the length of his nose and up the center of his forehead; two ran across his nose and were taped to his cheeks. With this tube, he breathed adequately, except when he contracted another infection, as he did again and again because his resistance was low. At such times a transparent plastic hood was placed over his head and warm vapor blown in. It leaked out under the bottom rim and rose in a small cloud around him.

Even with that assistance, however, he repeatedly came close to dying, entering the state that in hospitals is known as "coding." Sometimes it was a "slow code"—the heart rate slowed; he turned a dusky color because he was retaining too much carbon dioxide and not getting enough oxygen. Then he was quickly restored with a boost of oxygen-rich air, usually administered by "bagging," or hand-pumping with a balloonlike bag attached to a mask.

But, more than once, Chris sank into the state known as a "full-blown code"—cardiopulmonary arrest. Alarms sounded, a nurse rushed to tell a physician, and a resuscitation team crowded around him to administer full-scale intervention: artificial respiration with bag and mask, intubation, cardiac massage, and drugs including epinephrine (Adrenalin). Resuscitation is standard practice unless a baby clearly cannot be prevented from dying. Sometimes, when all hope is lost, a "no code" order is issued. This instructs staff to refrain from full-scale resuscitation if the patient is coding.

"Come on, Chris," a surgeon cajoled after one full-blown episode. "You'd better be good or I'll send you to outer space." Indeed, under his plastic bubble the baby looked ready to travel.

The ET breathing tube was not a long-range solution. The surgeons eventually decided to perform a tracheostomy: to make a surgical opening in the throat and insert a breathing tube. According to one of the surgeons, this simple procedure can help

7

normal babies do well. Fewer than half of the normal babies on whom tracheostomies have been performed have had problems, he said, and these often result from inept care and accidents.

Some physicians have reservations about the procedure. When prompted, one neonatologist remarked, "I feel so bad every time I send a baby home with a trach. Such a baby needs lots of care. You have to take care of the wound, pump the fluids out. He will not talk until the tube comes out, in a year or two—maybe. If the parents can't take care of such a baby, he might have to live in a hospital for a year."

Another doctor recalled babies who had died after undergoing tracheostomies as a result of a mucous plug or other obstruction. Sometimes it happened soon after the baby went home, some-times—even more tragically—a year or two later. A nurse worried about Chris's brother. Wouldn't he be tempted to drop something into that hole in the baby's throat?

Chris was now more than three months old. All this time Mariel had been coming to see him; a tiny woman of delicate beauty, she always wore a long dress and a smile. The smile was a mask she maintained as a courtesy to others, but it was like a reflection on a still lake. The slightest disturbance—a look, a question, a child crying—would break it, leaving the smooth face blank while a tear coursed downward like a drop of rain. Tears were stored behind the mask.

Mariel watched her baby, noticing how he arched his back, as if to escape from the terrible things being done to him. She ran her fingers over the scars on his neck and his chest, stroked his back, cringed with him as he was poked with more needles. She heard him tell her what the doctors could not hear: that his suffering was more than he could bear. One day she requested that he not be resuscitated the next time his heart or breathing failed. But the surgeons replied that that was impossible—if a straightforward remedy for a medical problem was available, they could not refuse to use it. Their failure to resuscitate Chris would be equivalent to their putting a pillow over his head.

Mariel spoke good English, but with a strong accent that some hospital personnel found hard to understand. At age thirty, she was still learning the ways of the country to which she had come a few years earlier. She was becoming confused. What was right? The doctors were fighting for her baby's life. How could she wish for his death? When she left the hospital she knew that Chris was asking to die. When she returned, talked to the doctors, and saw her son on an especially good day, she wanted him to live. When asked to sign a consent form for the tracheostomy, Mariel signed.

Did she have a choice? Could she have refused? When asked those questions, one surgeon replied, "I wouldn't operate on the trachea again. That would be hopeless. But this is strictly a minor mechanical problem. It is literally just putting in a little tube. We told the mother that if there were nothing we could do, we would not prolong his life. But we couldn't let him die without performing a tracheostomy because we couldn't know what his potential is."

He spoke from personal conviction but also with awareness of the law. Since the adoption of the 1984 "Baby Doe" regulations, physicians were no longer allowed much leeway in deciding when further aggressive treatment was undesirable. "The big difference now is in terms of whether you are withholding heroic treatment or standard care," another surgeon explained. "We would not propose another tracheal reconstruction or a heart/lung machine. There are limits within the law. But beyond that, it is difficult. In this case, the tracheostomy was standard. He could have lived a short time without it, but then he would have suffocated. With a standard procedure available, can we stand by and do nothing? Probably not."

Within that perspective, the surgeons would have felt obliged, under the law, to insist on the operation, even if the mother had refused consent. Medical institutions commonly ask for a court order when a parent objects to something physicians think they must do. When a child of Jehovah's Witnesses requires a blood transfusion, to which that sect objects, a court order to proceed is usually waiting at the hospital by the time the baby arrives. Unlike Chris Lew, most such children can be helped to get well and grow up normally. But since the Baby Doe controversy, there has been pressure to go further in denying parents a choice to refuse treatment. When parents refused surgery for a baby who was born with a severe form of intestinal atresia (congenital obstruction, often of the ileum) and Down's syndrome, one surgeon recalled, the hospital's lawyer went to court and the parents lost custody. The baby lived and was placed in an institution.

So Mariel Lew was not given a real choice at this point, because the surgeons felt compelled by law and ethics. And what of Chris's prospects, given the known facts? "We know he won't be normal," said the surgeon. "We don't know whether his deficit will be a little or a lot. The mother believes it will be a lot. We don't know."

Mariel came in just as the day-shift nurses were leaving and the swing shift was taking over. The X-ray technician was at Chris's bedside, adjusting the equipment for a chest radiogram. A nurse lifted him into sitting position and, steadying his wobbling head, held the child like a limp doll. At the last moment, just before the technician pushed the button, the nurse pulled the ET tube out of the new opening in Chris's throat. Mariel withdrew several feet, as did other adults in the room, this being required procedure to avoid radiation scatter. The other babies stayed where they were: the scatter is slight, but nursing and other staff are exposed much more often than patients. Of course, the nurse who was holding Chris stayed.

Mariel watched from the doorway, restraining herself against the pull toward her baby. Was the nurse gentle? Did she feel his suffering? Some nurses were more sensitive than others, she had observed. If she were a nurse, would she be able to do what they were now doing to this baby? He was so bruised and battered. There were the scars, the marks of repeated punctures on his arms and feet. The look in his eyes communicated suffering beyond Mariel's comprehension. Surely infants are innocent and born to joy, not suffering? He had been here more than a hundred days. She had come every day, only to stand helpless.

Later, she sat in the hospital cafeteria, speaking softly, evenly, as oblivious of the tears that flowed from her eyes as of the teacup before her. She had thought about what she wanted to say, and now the words came easily, without interruption.

"I ask, Whose fault? His parents'? God's? I ask, Why? Medically, religiously, humanly, it does not come together.

"Medically, they research what is wrong. They will fix the problem. So they continuously treat him even though he had a lot of suffering. A month ago, they were trying to put in an IV and I watched his face. He does not want to live, I thought. He is a baby, he cannot speak, but if you look close you can see. He would tell me, 'Why do you give me this much suffering? I cannot handle any more. Please let me go. Don't handle me again.' I touched him—very gently—and he was scared to death. But for almost an hour and a half they could not get in the IV. He cried. The nurse could not get it in and neither could the doctor when he arrived. The baby's vein moves; it is very difficult to find it and stick in the needle. The doctor said, 'Let's try later, he's too tired.' They tried later and finally got it in. I saw that and asked myself, Why?

"The next day he had trouble breathing. At the moment when he would have died the nurse took out the tube and paged a doctor. Chris had turned blue; his back arched; his head fell back. It was the moment of dying. When I saw that I prayed, 'Please God, bring him to You.' I prayed it. I expected that when the doctor came, he would tell me my baby had passed away. I would have kissed the doctor thank-you. But he came and said, 'He's okay.' I did not want to hear.

"Every time he does that—it has happened more than once or twice—I pray to God to take Chris to heaven. That is what I truly wanted. The doctor said he had brain damage. On the phone he told me that. If that is so, he cannot have a normal life. He will have no reason for life, for life is joyful and he will only suffer. I asked the doctor, 'Could you let him die?' He said no, because of the law.

"Then one night, at two A.M., I was awake and my mind was going. I called a nurse I know to tell her my story. She said, 'Ask for No Code, so he can go. They can stop the treatment.' So the next day I came to the hospital and told them, 'Please, No Code.' Still, they won't let him die.

"The doctor's duty is to save life. I don't want to complain. It's a very difficult job. Chris's operation was supposed to last six hours, but it lasted eight. They came out of the surgery room all sweaty and tired. That is why I cannot complain to them.

"And if I had known there would be so much suffering, would I have said no to the operation? I probably would have said yes, anyway. It is not a wise decision, I know, and that is what I do not understand in myself. When I see the baby suffer I pray to God to take him to heaven. But when I see him not suffering I pray, 'Thanks for his life.' I pray thanks for life and I pray for death. The prayers go in opposite directions, but I hope they will meet each other." Her hands rose from the table and formed a circle in front of her, then dropped into her lap.

"My husband does not come to the hospital," she said. "I brought a picture of Chris and said, 'He is like this now.' My husband put it on the table; he said nothing. Whatever the baby's condition, I have to accept it. I don't have a choice. Should I have a choice?"

A week later, there was a change in Mariel. She seemed to walk more firmly through the nursery. Chris was recovering from the tracheostomy and appeared to be feeling better. He had even smiled at her. He was growing. His first tooth was coming in.

"I have accepted now that there is no way I can help Chris," said his mother. "I will accept whatever happens to him. There is deafness; there is brain damage. He may live and have a very poor life. I am ready for that. Or he may die. I am also ready for that. I cannot help him."

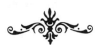

The Lew family's health plan coverage required that Chris be moved back to the hospital where he was born. As soon as the Stanford staff felt he could be taken care of there, the transfer was made. But he was brought back to Stanford a few weeks later for a bronchoscopy, an examination of the tracheal tube, and a laser treatment that helps widen that passage in babies whose stenosis was caused by a ventilator. Then he was returned to the original hospital, where he lived until he was seven and a half months old. His mother, who was working hard in the family's new business, no longer had to drive so far to visit him. She saw him improve to the point of seeming to enjoy rocking in a swing. She watched him play with his hands, sometimes folding them as if in prayer. His continued suffering led her to become a regular worshiper at the church she had occasionally attended.

Early in her son's first spring, just as the plum trees were beginning to flower, Mariel was told that Chris was ready to go home. She went to the hospital to learn how to care for him: to suction his excess fluids, to maintain the tube in his throat, to run the vaporizer that would supply the necessary warmth and moisture. Mariel was accompanied by her live-in housekeeper, who watched over the Lews' four- year-old son while his mother worked. But the older woman, who had come with the family from their home country, was so frightened by the tubes and electrical equipment surrounding the baby that she declared she would absolutely not tend to him. Mariel thought she would be able to persuade the housekeeper to change her mind once Chris was home.

On his third day home, Chris Lew died.

"He is gone. This morning," she said, her voice a flat whisper. Then, after a silence, "I did not know about the machine, the mister [vaporizer]. They said to change the water daily, but I did not know it could run out in three hours."

Mariel had brought Chris home at 3:00 A.M. on a Tuesday, two days earlier. A medical supply firm had delivered a vaporizer and suction pump that afternoon. The hospital order had not included a monitor. This had worried Mariel a little, and she thought perhaps she should get a bracelet that would rattle if Chris became agitated or distressed.

The vaporizer helped clear out the mucus and eased his breathing. But on Wednesday it had stopped working, so she'd called the supplier, who had a new one delivered. The baby kept having trouble, throwing up four times during the evening. She suctioned him repeatedly to make sure no mucous plug developed. By 1:00 A.M. Thursday morning, when he seemed to be all right, she had put him to bed. The vaporizer was working.

At 6:00 A.M. the housekeeper woke her: the baby was not breathing. He was cold, his back was arched, and he was still. He had thrust the nozzle of the vaporizer from his throat. Mariel looked at the tank and saw that the water level was below the intake point, which meant that only warm air had been blowing toward the hole in the baby's throat.

Mariel thought that Chris was dead, but she was not sure. She tried to suction him, but the tracheal tube was so plugged with mucus that she could not get the tube of the suction pump inside it. She held him. He seemed to sigh. She called the ambulance. At the hospital, she was told that Chris was dead.

Mariel sat on the rug in the middle of her living room, swaying slightly. "If I had taken care of him well he would still be alive," she lamented. "I did not know the water could run out so fast. When babies go home and are taken care of they live, don't they? It was my fault."

It did not comfort her to hear that other babies who had survived many months in the hospital had died after finally coming home. Her son had been judged ready to make the move. He had been her responsibility. She blamed herself.

"At Stanford they said he could live a long time. If he died so soon, why the operation? I should have said no. But even knowing what I now know, I perhaps would have said yes. I am so confused." She was silent for a long moment.

"What is this dying?" Mariel continued. "I do not know it. When he turned blue at the hospital, they bagged him and he came back. When he was paralyzed he seemed dead, but the doctor said he could hear, he could feel, he only could not move. This morning, how is it different? I think if I go to the hospital I will find him there, my baby, so much suffering and nobody listening to him, like Jesus, and no voice."

The telephone, on a small table next to a couch, rang, and she moved to answer. It was a doctor from the hospital that had sent Chris home, asking how he had died and telling her that an autopsy would have to be done.

"Using a knife, doctor? Will he have pain?"

She listened to the doctor's explanation.

"I don't want them to do that, doctor. You really have no choice?"

The law requires an autopsy when someone who dies at home has not been under a doctor's care for the previous twenty-four hours. If a doctor fails to order an autopsy, the coroner can demand one. However, it is possible to obtain a waiver when problems are well known, as they certainly were in this case.

"But what for? What for again?" asked Mariel. "Why still more cutting if he is dead? It is his body. Also my body. If he is not going to be alive again it is not necessary. Doctor, he seemed to be sleeping." She was pleading now. "How long has he been completely dead? Is there no way he can live again?"

She knew and she did not know. So many things had been strange and unlikely, had lacked referents in her own experience and had violated her intuitive judgment. She no longer knew what death meant or if pain stopped at death. What is a coroner, she asked, and what did he want with her baby's body? She wanted to bring him home so she could sit with him until the funeral. She called the physician. "Doctor, can I stay with him until he goes?" Again, she was told that was not possible.

"I must accept then, if I have no choice," she said. Once more she asked, "Should I have a choice?"

Two weeks before her baby son had died, Mariel again had a dream that she noted in her diary. It seemed to her not unconnected with the earlier dream about water, the worm, and the mouse, and with all that had occurred since.

This particular night, she had been unable to sleep. Her mind was at the hospital; she was tossing and turning. Eventually, so as not to disturb her husband with her restlessness, she took a quilt, went into the living room, and lay down on the floor, where she was now sitting. In her dream she was in a place that was either a court or a church. It resembled the traffic court where she had once had to appear about a ticket. Many people were milling about, waiting for something. Then a huge door opened and she was inside a space that was like a large auditorium. It was crowded with people all dressed in white robes except for one, her minister, who was wearing his usual black suit with clerical collar. He motioned to Mariel, and she took the seat to his right. The entire space was filled with music, though nobody was singing. It was like Christmas music, but Mariel had not heard it before.

She realized that Jesus was coming and looked up, expecting him to descend from on high. But then she saw that all eyes were turned in her direction, toward the place on her right, which was empty. As she, too, turned to look, a basket covered with a white blanket descended and settled beside her. She knew it was Chris and lifted the cover to look. But the basket was empty. No baby was inside; there was only light. She quickly covered the basket again.

No field in medicine is so compelling and so confusing, so wondrous and so disturbing, as neonatology, the care, study, and treatment of the newborn. In no other discipline is the reward for success so great and the price of failure so horrifying. Before 1960, the specialty did not exist. By the 1980s, it was the fastest growing subspeciality in pediatrics. The news media are full of its amazing achievements. Infants so small they fit into the palm of a hand survive. Birth defects that used to be fatal are microsurgically repaired. Even stillborn babies are sometimes brought back to life. Emotional public debates arise, and court battles are fought about choices of care and treatment in intensive care nurseries, about matters that actually involve a rather small number of people.

Why this high degree of public interest? In medicine, the only other specialty that stirs nearly as much excitement is cardiovascular surgery. Both the artificial heart and the artificially sustained baby touch something profound inside us. Both reach beyond the therapeutic into the mystical and raise questions about human nature and our cultural heritage.

Even more than cardiosurgery's artificial heart, neonatology is a terrain where values collide in unprecedented ways, uprooted

15

by new tools from ground where they had meaning. By looking at the ICN, we can gain insight into processes that shape the country and some of the ills that have befallen the body social: the predilection toward spectacular technological achievements in crisis and the neglect of much simpler, less costly, and more effective possibilities of averting these crises; the breakdown of trust as specialization renders people incomprehensible to each other; the preoccupation with goals that blinds us to the means. We can see how technology becomes an imperative, a driving force that obscures the purpose for which it was devised. We can also see the distance that grows between human actions and common sense when the mind is captured by technology. A close look at the workings of neonatology allows us to perceive these problems, which exist throughout society, even while we continue to admire and be amazed.

The advances of neonatology and the related field of perinatology (high-risk obstetrics) across biological boundaries stir an excitement not unlike that generated by the space program in the early 1960s. There is a sense of unlimited possibilities.

As in preceding decades astronauts opened new vistas beyond the earth, so now medical scientists, penetrating the limits of birth, are creating new opportunities for seizing control over our biological development. We can see inside the womb and watch the sacred process of an individual human life's beginning. We can intervene and choose.

However, hand in hand with this progress run its side effects, threatening to trip it and send it crashing into a nightmarish domain where, as in George Orwell's *1984*, things become the opposite of what they were intended to be. In the intensive care nursery, where the dramas of neonatology unfold, equipment designed to be therapeutic can turn into machinery for torture. Saving life can mean prolonged dying. Babies are "saved" only to be confined to institutions as total care patients, while their families are destroyed by the "rescue." The burden of choice is as great as its potential.

Some people try to understand this growing tension between opposites by saying that we have usurped the prerogative of God or nature or fate. They argue that we have arrogated unto ourselves decision-making powers that belong elsewhere and, in so doing, are guilty of hubris, the original sin of the Garden of Eden—wanting to be like gods (Genesis 3:5). Typically, this charge is leveled against physicians, who, more than the members of any other profession, are often accused of playing God. It may be that the decisions of politicians, nuclear scientists, military leaders, and economists (among others) are as momentous for human destiny and the life of the cosmos as any made by physicians. Yet, somehow, physicians alone seem to be identified as a group guilty of appropriating powers that are properly the divine prerogative.

It is interesting to ask why physicians should be singled out, and labeled haughty, among all those who, one way or another, wield power in the world. Perhaps it is because the decisions doctors make affect identifiable, individual lives, whereas others' decisions affect people more generally and are usually issued anonymously. Our culture often accords value and respect to the individual at the expense of the common good.

Perhaps it is because of the value we place on the individual that physicians are accused of playing God. However, it may also be that many of us, at one time or another, want them to do so. Any of us who have confronted an intractable health problem, one we have failed to alleviate by our most strenuous efforts—such as exercise, nutrition, stress reduction, and meditation—know that, having done all we could do to restore the status quo ante, we yearn for someone in a white coat. Our expectation that wellness is the norm, that disease and death are not part of the human condition, leads us to fantasize that doctors will do what we cannot do for ourselves and magically put right what has gone wrong. Sometimes they can.

Be that as it may, there is another way to look at the decisions doctors make at the beginning of a life. It is to recognize that human beings are endowed by the Creator with freedom and responsibility and that making decisions is thus expressive, not necessarily of hubris, but of the very essence of the humanum. We are free, using our God-given brains, to invent new modalities for preserving or extending life and to decide when, or when not, to apply them. We are also responsible for the choices we make, and must be willing to live with them, without displacing blame or praise onto others.

Of the two alternatives regarding our power to intervene in what Darwin called the process of natural selection, we prefer the second. Freedom and responsibility, rather than usurpation of a divine prerogative, are at the heart of the matter; the power to choose is indicative not of hubris, but of the awesome weight of striving to become fully and truly human.

17

The responsibility for the choices we are free to make increases, almost from year to year, largely because of expansion in the domains of technology, economics, and the law. At a pace so rapid that it is almost impossible to keep up with, let alone get ahead of, technology—particularly medical technology—proliferates. Tools and techniques are invented and applied, not only in neonatology but in such esoteric and diverse areas as in vitro fertilization and embryo implantation, the transplantation of organs across the boundary of species, angioplasty, and mechanical heart implantations. Typically, the technology is developed and applied before any of us—let alone those who first decide to use it—have had time to consider the moral ramifications, the ethical implications, of what is being done. Only after the fact, and sometimes in a desperate game of "catch up," do we begin to reckon with the consequences of our decisions, by which time it is usually too late to reverse the thrust of technology in the area that concerns us.

At the same time, medical expenditures in the United States have been rising at a rate four times that of the general rate of inflation, and twice that of the consumer price index, without any dramatic or even discernible improvement in our general health or well-being as compared with people in nations where the technology is equal to, but the expenditures for medical care are less than, ours. Now that we have become aware of the need to contain, if not curtail, expenditures for medical care by means of various cost containment systems, economic considerations inevitably begin to enter what once were thought to be purely medical decisions. Does society approve of spending $120,000 to "rescue" a premature, very low-birth-weight infant when the same amount, if used to provide preventive medical and social care for pregnant women, could obviate the need for intensive care for many more infants? If it costs $120,000 to rescue such a premature, very low-birth-weight infant, is it ever right, on economic grounds, to discontinue an aggressive course of therapy already begun, or to refuse to escalate it? These are but some of the questions forced on us by the runaway costs of medical care. Making decisions at the threshold of life is complicated and difficult.

Choices are also becoming more onerous because of the increasing intrusion by courts and the federal government into what used to be an arena occupied almost exclusively by physicians, nurses, and parents. No longer may decisions be made solely by the principals involved. Now laws and regulations prescribe aggressive treatment for all newborns except those in a fairly circumscribed category in which aggressive treatment would in any case be futile, as when a baby's problems—neurological, physiological, or both—are so severe that only extremely short-term survival is possible.

The law, however, is uninformed on the realities of intensive care. It fails to take account of the fact that intensive care is not a direct treatment but a powerful, violent, and risky interim medical measure. A physician who institutes it takes on the responsibility of following through, as he does with any medical measure. If the likelihood of recovery is small, the risks of intensive care interventions become unreasonable. The burden of pain they impose on the patient is no longer justifiable under the physician's commitment to the principle *Primum non nocere:* Above all, do no harm.

With legal constraints in place, inappropriate, and likely to multiply, making decisions about withholding or withdrawing aggressive technology for what is popularly called "quality of life" considerations becomes increasingly difficult. Those who formerly bore the lonely burden of making such decisions—neonatologists, nurses, and parents—now find their freedom inhibited and their responsibility diminished. They are confronted by an additional moral dilemma: whether to obey the courts or their own conscience.

So medical caregivers must find ways to use their freedom and responsibility, within the opportunities and constraints created by technological, economic, and legal expansion, to benefit the infants and families they serve.

Underlying the various factors that contribute, directly or indirectly, to the difficulty of decision making in the newborn (as well as other) intensive care units is a societal inability to accept death as part of life. Ours is a death-denying culture. Youthfulness, vitality, and outward beauty are steadily portrayed as the norm; to be aging, impotent, and manifestly in a state of decline that will inevitably end in death is not part of the popular scenario. The pivotal events of the life cycle—birth, sickness, suffering, aging, and death—no longer take place in the home. Children are insulated from their frequently harsh reality. This phenomenon, perhaps more than any other, underlies our unease and even incompetence in choosing who should live and who should die. For if there is indeed a powerful death-denying tendency in our culture, to accept the inexorability of finitude, of mortality, and of the conditional nature of our existence, is surely beyond us. There will be times, therefore, when we opt for what we think is life, but in fact is no more than mere physical existence, without anything remotely approaching those capacities which make life good, meaningful, rich, and full. Indeed, this is perhaps the ultimate pathos.

Primum non nocere, which has been basic to the physician's commitment since the time of Hippocrates, has served as a restraint against overzealousness in the practice of a hazardous art. (In the past, of course, a doctor had only comfort to offer for conditions that are now routinely treatable.) All medical interventions inflict some measure of harm on patients. But generally speaking, such harm caused, for example, by sticking needles into the body, cutting it open, irradiating it, or poisoning it with chemotherapy, is thought to be justified by the expected benefits of the interventions. The damage done is usually reckoned to be slight by comparison with the large, hoped-for compensatory gains.

However, it is difficult to apply this calculation in the high-risk nursery. For one thing, we cannot imagine what infants experience during the most routine interventions— withdrawal of blood samples, intravenous injections, intubation, ventilation, or induced paralysis to conserve their energies, for example. What an adult perceives as routine may be traumatic for a newborn. For another, our interventions, marvels of technology, may condemn infants who would have died without them to exist in a twilight zone of physical disability and neurological deficit, or both, which their rescuers cannot adequately comprehend. There is a fine line between salvaging high-risk infants and harming them—not merely temporarily but permanently. A line must be drawn beyond which "routine" interventions can produce more harm than good. Drawing that line, perceiving that point, is admittedly difficult and sometimes impossible. In this book we tell of babies and families who have ultimately benefited from the pain inflicted on them. We also tell of others for whom the line was drawn mistakenly, the point passed without being perceived, so that infants and families were irreparably harmed by the well-intentioned interventions of those who made decisions on their behalf.

It is true that neonatal intensive care has, in fact, decreased infant mortality. However, it must be noted that the major factor associated with infant mortality is prematurity, and that the rate of prematurity has remained virtually the same for two decades.

In Sweden, the premature birth rate is half that of the United States. This can be partly explained by the fact that Sweden has addressed some of the primary problems contributing to prematurity: adverse socioeconomic conditions faced by pregnant women—poor housing, bad nutrition, inadequate prenatal medical care.[1] The emphasis in the United States has been on rescuing low-birth-weight infants from death *after* birth, at much greater cost and by means of highly sophisticated technology. Why? Why has this country not taken Sweden's approach? In part, the American choice reflects a national fascination with technology and acute medical care. It also highlights a national preference for quick, rather than slow, solutions to problems. In part, it perhaps also reflects an indifference to the poor. In a land where those who have made it to the top tend to claim there is unlimited opportunity for all, the facile notion exists that those who have not made it have only themselves to blame. Ameliorating their adverse socioeconomic conditions goes against the grain. It is easier to use technology in the nursery.

Neonatology has parents confused, doctors and nurses anguished, hospitals on the defensive, politicians and religious groups in the fray. It has brought philosophers into major medical centers to help those who must grope their way through the enormously difficult moral issues that have been raised. As in other fields where technology has developed far faster than society's comprehension of its meaning and our ability to deal with the consequences (nuclear energy and recombinant DNA research, for instance), the question is, Are we ready to wield this new power for the sake of enhancing life? Is there a wise sorcerer in charge in key places or are there only ambitious sorcerer's apprentices, smart but lacking in wisdom and therefore dangerous?

The new choices created by technology are difficult in acute care medicine as a whole, but they are especially so in the case of newborns, because they cannot speak for themselves and because the stakes are so high. For an elderly patient, a few more years of life are involved; for an infant there could be three score and ten.

Who shall choose when heroic measures are used on an infant? How much weight shall be given to the views of the doctors, the parents? What is the best interest of a child who faces only a minimal chance at life and a major probability of extreme disabilities? When shall the choice be made? On what grounds? How shall the goal of saving life be weighed against the impulse for compassion?

21

These major questions are being debated. They have become more urgent as neonatology has continued to push back the frontier of viability. There is no longer a clear distinction between a marginally viable baby and a late fetus, for instance, which creates an anomaly: a fetus can legally be aborted up to twenty-four weeks' gestation in some states, yet in the same hospital, in the ICN, heroic measures are used to keep twenty-four-week fetus/babies alive, sometimes against the parents' wishes.

The sophisticated life-support technology that has created the necessity for choice sometimes preempts that choice. In the midst of the confusion of values, it dictates its use by its very existence, sometimes—like a sorcerer's power in the hands of his apprentice—with monstrous consequences.

The broad philosophical questions raised by this technology are manifest in specific experiences in the ICN, particularly with infants who are very sick or impaired. Only through understanding such experiences— each unique and a composite of many interactions—can the ethical issues in neonatology be truly understood.

The issues as they appear from within the nursery are not what they seem from without. The doctors' problem is not what those lacking ICN experience believe it to be. They do not sit down at any point to weigh whether a life is "worth" saving. That is not how the problem presents itself. Their task in borderline cases is to decide whether, in applying or continuing aggressive life support, they would be working for their patients' benefit or doing harm.

Few doctors, if any, would use all the tools at their disposal to keep alive infants whom they know to be so injured that they have no chance of being autonomous, knowing self, sharing in the life of a community. Most would see aggressive intervention in such instances as a violation of the physician's creed, "Do no harm."

Certainty is rare in medicine. Statistics show that infants with various problems are at various degrees of risk for serious disability. These statistics are often inadequate, and they keep changing. Before 1980, infants of 600 grams (1 lb. 5 oz.), for instance, hardly ever survived, so it is impossible to know how those now surviving will do as they grow. New therapies keep altering the probabilities. Intracranial hemorrhage used to be an almost sure sign of neurological damage in premature infants. Then, ultrasound and electroencephalogram tests showed that among very low-birth-weight infants such bleeds were far more common than had been believed and that many survived them without such damage. At the same time, new treatment techniques have considerably diminished the risk, even with more serious bleeds. But long-term effects remain largely unknown because the improvements are so recent.

Solid statistical data about outcome helps, but it does not relieve a physician of the burden of choice. Statistics show only degrees of risk for categories of infants: babies with worst-case EEG tests, worst-case brain bleeds, chronic lung disease; babies born at a certain birth weight or within a particular gestational age range. It may be possible to look at a baby and say what the degree of risk might be for that infant. But everyone knows of "miracle" babies who defied statistical probability. So physicians read statistics and weigh them differently, according to personal values and experience.

Dr. David K. Stevenson, associate director of nurseries at Stanford University Medical Center, points out that statistics give data only about populations, not individuals. A particular baby may prove to be the exception. Therefore, he maintains, "If you use only categories to make decisions, you assume responsibility for having, essentially, executed a normal person some of the time."

His is one point of view on the matter. Some of his colleagues have other perspectives. One points out that, since there are no certainties in medicine, doctors are always forced to use their best judgment within uncertainty. It is irresponsible to ignore facts and risks, he says. The price of ignoring probability is the survival of babies who did not beat the odds, many of whom are condemned to life rather than saved. These babies would have died if a physician had not used heroic measures to keep them alive. By trying to rescue them, physicians may be preventing a release from torment.

"We are now interfering with death and we have no business doing that," observed the medical director of an institution for the severely disabled, standing in a room full of children sustained by tracheostomies, gastrostomies, and nasogastric feeding pumps. "Modern medicine has created a new element—a living death. It goes on for many years. For parents, the loss of a child through death is, at least, final. It is far more difficult for them to adjust to a living death."

Most physicians try to share the burden of decision making with colleagues, nurses, and especially with parents. Sometimes, however, the parents are not really heard because a vast gulf in interest, experience, and perception separates them from doctors.

In the thick folders that contain Chris Lew's medical history, no space is provided for the entry of his mother's dreams. The surgeons continued to consider the tracheal reconstruction a success. They were pleased that the part of the windpipe they had restructured had healed and looked normal. But in view of the complications of the treatment, they thought that in a similar situation they might do a tracheostomy sooner.

Did Mariel Lew share in the physicians' choices regarding Chris? Should she have had more options? What shaped the surgeons' decisions regarding her infant? What part did research interest play and how did it affect their judgment of what was best for Chris and his family? Did the Baby Doe regulations prevent the surgeons from letting Chris die?

The issue of therapy versus research presents itself in all acute care medicine, not only in the nursery. The commitment to do no harm vies with other motivations—the curiosity of the scientist, the desire to help future patients, personal ambition, and the desire to publish. Federal regulations are a relatively new additional factor predisposing toward intervention when the alternative is certain death, especially in research hospitals. By requiring that standard treatment not be withheld, they help to reinforce the other motivations for zealousness in treatment.

Did Mariel Lew have a choice? The surgeons indicated that she did not at the time she was asked to sign a consent form for the tracheostomy. She could have refused the original operation, the tracheoplasty. Certainly she was told that the chance of success was slim. Also certainly, she did not understand what form "success" could take. Yet, after the death of her child, she said that even if she had known what suffering would follow, she might have agreed. She would have gone for the dim gleam of hope. Some physicians believe that to offer a choice when the alternative is certain death is, in itself, coercive to parents.

What about Mariel Lew's requests that her baby not be resuscitated? The surgeons felt compelled, by law and their own ethics. They also said that the case was made especially difficult, from their point of view, by the mother's inconsistency: she had wavered in her expressed desire that the baby be allowed to die.

Did the surgeons understand the mother's intention accurately? Another nursery staffer, who was in frequent contact with Mariel Lew, said it was "her theme from the beginning" that Chris wanted to and should be allowed to die.

Even assuming she did waver—what mother would not, meeting her child's gaze, his conscious recognition, seeing one of his rare smiles? How did such wavering relate to the way the physicians informed her of her child's state?

Some close observers maintain that a doctor has the power to obtain a parent's agreement to any course of treatment, that the parent is always swayed by the manner in which the doctor in charge presents the choice. Few parents have either the broad medical knowledge or the emotional detachment to hold to an agenda that opposes that of the doctors, especially if they choose against heroic measures.

In the case of Chris Lew, the surgeons appeared committed to continuing to treat aggressively. One of them remarked, reproachfully, that "the mother's problem" was her unwillingness to accept a retarded baby.

Should parents have more choice? Should their personal values and religious and cultural background be considered? Physicians in the Stanford nursery have slight experience with the diverse cultures their patient populations represent. In many cultures—as in the United States until recently—a baby born with severe disabilities was deemed a baby unequipped to live. The right course with such babies was to "put them down": wrap them warmly but do nothing extraordinary either to save them or to help them expire.

Heroic measures are the final effort. The definition of *heroic* changes with time and circumstance. But the option of avoiding extraordinary treatment has been seriously narrowed in recent court decisions. In *Baby Doe,* the parents allowed a Down's syndrome infant to die by refusing to permit surgery that would have enabled him to take in food. The case raised much indignation and became a stepping-stone toward federal regulations that would compel surgery in similar cases. Before *Baby Doe,* many doctors took family circumstances into account when they quietly and privately made decisions about Down's syndrome babies.

In the subsequent *Baby Jane Doe* case, the parents of a more seriously defective infant, with spina bifida (congenital cleft of the vertebral column) and other complications, opted not for withdrawal of care but for the less aggressive of two options. They did not, as was argued by those who intruded into the matter, choose death. They selected the less violent medical course, which would not force life on their baby if she was not prepared to live. After a right-to-life attorney who heard about the case sued the hospital to force aggressive treatment, a guardian was appointed to ascertain and represent the baby's best interest. He found the original therapeutic course acceptable. But the story became further entangled when the White House intervened on the right-to-life attorney's side.

Then a federal law narrowing physicians' options for defective newborns was passed. However, as of 1985, this law was still open to wide interpretation and was being read in different ways. What are options for some may not be for others. To a degree, seeing options is related to insight, courage, and attention.

Clearly, Mariel Lew felt she had no choice. So did many other parents who—painfully, and torn by doubt and self-reproach—have asked doctors to let their babies go and were refused. The bias toward aggressive treatment, and the small measure of parental choice within the medical system, have been documented in other reports. However, when parents request the reverse—when physicians believe extraordinary measures are inadvisable but parents ask them to do all they can for their baby—the parental plea is far more likely to be heeded, even honored as a command. The physician still chooses.

The intensive care nursery is an arena of creative conflict. New questions arise from new scientific discoveries, compelling a shift in thinking that affects far more than the infant patients and their families.

For a doctor who has to make a decision about a borderline baby, a commitment to saving life is not enough, because court cases have already been argued on the premise that life can be "wrongful." A constitutional perspective is not enough, for it comes up against the maxim "Above all, do no harm." To recognize someone's rights and to inflict a painful life on a person are not the same. In law, society has decided that it is better for many guilty people go free lest one innocent man be convicted. This is a basic principle, embedded in the Constitution. But if the extreme civil libertarian approach is brought to neonatology—the fear of "executing a normal person" echoes the legal principle—it is not a question of freeing guilty people that is involved, but of other innocents—infants unequipped for life—being sentenced to survival.

The ICN is a manifestation of our society. It reflects what we are: people who love to tinker and sometimes, in taking things apart and putting them together again in new ways, lose our sense of the whole; who hold that each human being is endowed with certain inalienable rights but sometimes fail to take account of the fact that everything and everyone exists in relationship. We love new frontiers and keep searching for new worlds to discover or conquer, but often fail to get fully acquainted with the place where we live. It is conceivable that someday babies will be manufactured to order in artificial wombs, to be picked up nine months later, like new automobiles. At the same time it is possible that, through science and our native gifts, we will find the way to a new appreciation of the sacredness and mystery of life. The ICN is a place where we can assess our gains and, by looking closely, take note of what we have sacrificed in the bargain.

As a microbiologist looks at arrangements of molecules, seeking to detect something more about the functioning of organisms of which they are a part, so we can look at one particular ICN and the lives that are touched by it and thereby, perhaps, understand some of the questions facing both this area of medicine and, in a larger sense, all of society.

We have chosen to focus on marginally viable babies because that is where the issues on the frontier of neonatology are presented most sharply. These babies comprise a small percentage of those who pass through the ICN, but they are important in the way that the people who live on in constitutional law are important—Brown in *Brown v. Board of Education*, the case that led to outlawing segregation in schools; Roe in *Roe v. Wade*, which established wide rights to abortion. They are the snags in the current that can change the course of a stream. They are the ones doctors remember long after they have forgotten 90 percent or more of the babies who have gone on to lead normal, healthy lives, thanks in part to what medicine was able to do for them. These are the babies who raise the issues.

The history of ethical problems in neonatology can, in fact, be charted with the names of babies the way English history used to be charted for grade school students by the names of kings: David the Bubble Boy, who was born without an immune system and lived his twelve years confined within a plastic container that separated him from all other life; Baby Doe and Baby Jane Doe; Baby

Fae, in whom a baboon heart was implanted; Babies A through G, the septuplets born to Patricia Frustaci after she took a fertility drug. While the vast majority of some two hundred thousand infants who pass through some six hundred intensive care nurseries in the United States annually grow up to be normal citizens and never make news, these babies are historical markers.

The infants described in this book were known only to their families and friends and the people at Stanford University Medical Center. Almost all were born on the threshold of viability, except for a few who were beyond the reach of medical arts. Some were "miracle" babies who survived and went on to their families despite heavy odds. Some died. Some lingered for many months and drifted toward a cloudy future. The particulars of their lives are molecules from which the big issues are composed.

CHAPTER TWO

From the Carnival Circuit to High-Tech Circuitry

One of the most popular attractions at the Berlin Exposition of 1896 was Professor Pierre-Constant Budin's child hatchery (Kinderbrutanstalt), featuring six incubators containing premature babies. Not even the sky rides or the Congolese village attracted such crowds. People paid one German mark for a look.

Dr. Budin, a physician from Paris, later became known as the father of neonatology. He was using the Berlin fair to spread the word about the technique that he and his teacher, Professor Etienne Tarnier, had developed to help premature infants survive. Having observed a correlation between the ability of premature infants to maintain normal body temperature and their rate of survival, Dr. Tarnier had commissioned a zookeeper to design an incubator, patterned after one used with chicks, that provided heated air, additional humidity, and temperature monitoring for human babies. Dr. Budin was getting good results with this predecessor of the modern isolette in Paris, but, "In the world of science, nothing really counted in those days until it had received German approval," according to a later account.[1] So Dr.Budin sent an assistant, Martin Couney, to exhibit six of the incubators, containing babies lent for the occasion by the Berlin Charité Hospital. Since the babies were not expected to live, the risk was judged acceptable.

The infants survived the fair, and the exhibit's success launched Dr. Couney on an international circuit. He was invited to bring the display to the huge Victorian Exposition the following year in London and accepted. When the British would not lend infants from their hospitals, Dr. Budin arranged for him to import babies from France in three laundry baskets, using a heating system of hot water bottles under pillows. After that Dr. Couney proceeded to Paris and, with missionary zeal, continued the show for another thirty-nine years in North America, at trade fairs and expositions throughout the United States, and even in South America, becoming famous as the "incubator doctor." Because he offered free care and a chance at survival, parents proved willing to lend him their frail newborns. Eventually he set up a permanent exhibit in New York's Coney Island, but continued to travel. At the 1933–1934 Century of Progress Exposition in Chicago, his show was next to that of Sally Rand, the fan dancer, and was almost as popular.

Thousands of premature infants had experienced life's beginning as fair displays by the time Dr. Couney died in 1952. The success of the shows attracted imitators, provoking warnings and criticism in the pages of medical journals. But Dr. Budin's original purpose was realized: use of incubators spread. And when, in 1923, Dr. Julius Hess opened the first American premature baby nursery at Sarah Morris Hospital in Chicago, it was to some extent the result of his meeting Dr. Couney.

Meanwhile, even as his former associate was making the carnival circuit, Dr. Budin continued to write about and study the development of newborn infants. He opened special units for preterm babies at two Paris hospitals, the Maternité of Port Royal and the Clinique Tarnier, which became leading centers for clinical research and teaching.

By and large, however, medical investigators showed little interest in newborn infants until the mid-1960s. In the early part of this century, infants were not generally deemed the proper concern of physicians until they had survived their first month, or even until after they had been weaned. Almost all women gave birth at home. Only the poor and homeless tended to seek asylum in hospitals.

Then a drastic change in birthing practices occurred. By the 1920s, birth had ceased to be primarily a family event and became a medical procedure, which it has, to a large extent, continued to be in this country despite a movement in recent years toward natural childbirth. Physicians viewed every birth as a dangerous process that could lead to a variety of ills, including tears in a woman's perineum, convulsions, sepsis, and deformed pelvis. To avert trouble, they intervened routinely. Hospital births became the standard for urban families. The delivering woman became a patient.

How and why this perspective developed in this country— and not, for instance, in Scandinavian countries—has been the subject of several interesting inquiries by medical anthropologists and others. To delve into the question would shed light on current treatment of newborns but is beyond the scope of this work. Suffice it to say that within the attitude that birth was a dangerous process needing medical aid, the hospital seemed safer than the home.

An influential advocate of routine medical intervention into the process of birth was Dr. Joseph B. DeLee of Chicago. In a 1920 article, "The Prophylactic Forceps Operation," published in the *American Journal of Obstetrics and Gynecology,* he advised that episiotomies be standard practice and that forceps be used to lift out the infant's head and extract the placenta. The mother would be sedated while her cervix dilated, given ether before the skin and muscles in her perineum were cut, then ergot or a derivative to contract the uterus. By the 1930s, this procedure had been adopted as routine in many hospitals in the United States. Later, critics would suggest that the tearing of the perineum might have been a consequence of placing women on their backs, with legs in stirrups, during delivery.[2]

The shift to hospital deliveries set childbirth in the United States on a course for increasing medical intervention, to the point that women felt they had to give themselves over to the doctors and were unable to accomplish on their own something they and other mammals had been doing since the species began.

The complete institutionalization of childbirth did not, however, take place until recently. As late as the 1940s, many women were still delivering at home. Premature babies were sometimes taken to hospitals where they were kept in strict isolation, for the sake of avoiding infection, and parents were excluded. Little was known about these babies' needs and development.

In the 1930s, oxygen-enriched air began to be used systematically to help babies with respiratory problems. In the 1940s, the practice of blowing 100 percent oxygen into incubators became widespread. The result was an early example of the iatrogenic (treatment-induced) problem that would plague physicians in ever new forms as they advanced in this area: an intervention that alleviated one problem created another. The eyes of many infants were injured by a condition called retrolental fibroplasia (RLF) or retinopathy of prematurity, a condition in which the retina becomes damaged and, in the most severe stage, detached, causing visual impairment. This condition, previously unknown, appeared two years after the use of oxygen was begun, and by the 1950s it was the leading cause of blindness in children. Overzealous treatment was at least in part to blame. Later it was discovered that the survival rate of preterm infants routinely treated with oxygen was no different from that of preemies who had not been treated. Most of the treatment was probably unnecessary.[3]

Beyond incubation, isolation, oxygen, and gavage feeding (through tubes from the nose or mouth into the stomach), however, there was little special treatment available for premature infants and little research interest. In 1959, most large medical centers had one pediatrician who specialized in the newborn, but that was not an exclusive responsibility. At Stanford, Dr. Louis Gluck took care of the newborns and worked in the general pediatric ward. Dr. Philip Sunshine, as a resident and later as a fellow, worked with newborns, as well as with older children who suffered from gastrointestinal diseases. Both became leaders in the field that, until 1960, did not even have its name, neonatology.

In the 1960s, several developments combined to launch the new medical specialty and spur its growth, the death of President John F. Kennedy's premature baby not the least among them. President Kennedy's second son, born in 1963, about a month early, died of hyaline membrane disease, which is now called respiratory distress syndrome (RDS).

Dr. Sunshine believes that this single event was probably more influential than any other: "People then focused on this problem, since it had affected the President's baby. A lot of articles were written about hyaline membrane disease, about what could be done about it, and government money began to pour in. And that was really the impetus for the establishment of ICNs."

In 1956, Phil Sunshine had come from Denver for a year's pediatrics residency at Stanford, largely because he expected to be drafted and hoped to postpone that eventuality by seeking additional training. His intention was eventually to set up a family practice in a small town in Colorado. After a year, he entered the navy as a pediatrician. But though he was then eligible to begin practice, he did not meet his own requirement for a children's doctor: he was still unmarried and had no children. So he returned to Stanford to research gastrointestinal development, which was to become a lifetime interest. Under Dr. Gluck's influence, he became aware of how little was known about newborns and how much one could learn by careful observation.

So he never left Stanford to set up a family practice but went on to become the director of nurseries, a leading researcher on preterm infant nutrition, one of the first advocates of his day for the use of mother's milk, and an innovator in ICN management. He also more than met his own standard for pediatric practice by fathering five children. Looking back on his life after twenty-five years of medical practice, he found it "unbelievably gratifying."

Of the three neonatologists who took turns directing the Stanford ICN until mid-1985, when a fourth, Dr. William Benitz, joined the team, Dr. Sunshine has the most comfortable presence. His round face and kind eyes fit his name. Parents who arrive in a state of shock and terror are grateful for the reassurance he conveys. Those who work with him trust his experience and empathy.

Dr. Sunshine watched intensive care nurseries mushroom around the country and keep proliferating, even to excess. They grew out of premature infant nurseries, which had been in existence here and there since 1923, but were heavily regulated and primarily designed for infants needing extra time in an incubator; sick babies went into the pediatrics ward. But when, in the late 1960s, physicians began to work more and more with sick premature and other newborns, and with infants with surgical problems, the need for separate facilities became apparent. To get around the licensing restrictions governing premature infant nurseries, Dr. Sunshine recalled, pediatricians called them intensive care nurseries. "And that changed the way they took care of babies. It was the beginning of neonatology, as far as I'm concerned," Dr. Sunshine added. The nurseries became the arena for clinical research and invited postgraduate work on their populations.

The entry of the March of Dimes Foundation into this field further stimulated its development. The foundation's money had been going into polio research, but that disease had been vanquished and birth defects were chosen as the new target. The March of Dimes began to provide money to develop nurseries and follow-up clinics and for research.

As medical interest in sick newborns grew, insurance companies were encouraged to start covering them. Until then, coverage had begun only when an infant had come home from the hospital and was two to six weeks old. In 1976, Dr. Leo Bell, a private practitioner in San Mateo and a member of the California Medical Association's house of delegates, led a move to get the CMA to mandate coverage from day one, then persuaded State Assemblywoman Yvonne Braithwaite-Burke of Los Angeles to sponsor legislation to that effect. With a push from the medical society, the bill was passed and signed into law by Governor Ronald Reagan.[4] California became the first state to require coverage of newborn intensive care. Within the next three years, every state imposed this requirement.

Meanwhile, the beginning of Medicare and federal reimbursement to hospitals for the costly nursery service further stimulated the growth of neonatology. At that time, technology was not very far advanced and nobody could foresee what the costs would grow to be, or how far life saving could extend.

Stanford was the first facility to get a grant from the National Institutes of Health (NIH) for a premature infant research center. "Dr. Norman Kretchmer, the chairman of the department of pediatrics at that time, was very much involved in NIH activities and he kept saying that they should study preemies," recalled Dr. Sunshine. "Finally convinced, they said, 'Okay, if you can write a grant in three weeks we'll do it.' So we wrote one and they approved it."

The NIH was interested partly because the infant mortality rate in the United States was much higher than in other developed countries, and because the infant mortality rates of other countries were decreasing rapidly. This country ranked eleventh in the world in 1960, with an infant mortality rate of twenty-six per thousand, behind Japan and several European nations, including Norway and East Germany. The major cause of newborn deaths is low birth weight, which results from prematurity or growth retardation in the uterus. The Stanford group had persuaded NIH that this situation called for a center dedicated to research on the growth and development of preterm infants.

It was logical that any effort to decrease the infant death rate should relate to low birth weight. But this logic did not dictate concentration on neonatal intensive care. Prevention was an alternative, one that might have been far more humane and cost-effective. However, although efforts in that direction were made, the major national investment went toward dealing with the results of prematurity, the frail fetuses or babies.

The NIH-funded Premature Infant Research Center at Stanford began in 1962 as a separate entity from the nursery, with its own nursing staff. Later, the infants were moved into the ICN population at large, and the former research unit came to be known simply as Room One.

Use of a respirator for newborn infants began in several places at about the same time. It had been tried earlier in South Africa for infants with tetanus. A doctor in Chicago had ventilated an infant with hyaline membrane disease with a tracheostomy in place. In 1961 several research hospitals, including Vanderbilt Medical Center in Nashville and Toronto Children's Hospital, began to try this form of life support with newborns, using different techniques. The first baby was put on a ventilator at Stanford in 1962, over Dr. Sunshine's protest. "We didn't think it was a good thing to do," he said. "A more senior person and I had talked about it. But two very bright residents and an anesthesiologist decided to try it with a preemie who was actually dying, hypotensive, and in respiratory failure. She weighed around four pounds—we would now consider her a large preemie—but she had serious hyaline membrane disease. Her mother was a diabetic and this was really her only chance to have a live baby. That baby, now twenty-two years old, is doing fairly well. She lives with her father; her mother has died. She has some neurological and intellectual impairment, but she is not considered mentally retarded according to the standard that a person with an IQ of at least 80 is not so classified."

Dr. Sunshine paused. The question of outcome was then and would continue to be troublesome, and all too often, statistical manipulation could mask its meaning. "It used to be that you were considered mentally retarded if your IQ was below 90," he said. "Then millions of kids were turned normal when the definition was changed to below 80." This did not, of course, alter the fact that at age twenty-two, Stanford's first ventilator survivor was unable to care for herself without help.

"We had a lot of questions: Are we keeping alive babies who should not be? Are we going to end up with some horribly damaged infants? It was a concern we had for about three years," continued Dr. Sunshine. "But by the end of that year we had tremendous experience. We selected babies—usually over 1500 gram birth weight—with very low pH factors [whose blood was very acidic because of decreased ventilation and ability to eliminate carbon dioxide]. We had no mechanism for measuring Po_2 [the oxygen tension in the blood] at the time. If we saw a baby becoming apneic [breathing irregularly], stopping breathing, or just horribly cyanotic [bluish from oxygen deprivation], we would put the baby on the ventilator. We did not know what pressures to use, or what kind of rates, and we could only control oxygen at three different concentrations—room air [21 percent], 40 percent and 100 percent. There were no gradations.

"It was a fly-by-night operation. But then we noticed that what we needed to do was keep the baby breathing for two or three days and then let the baby take over. If it required 100 percent oxygen for more than two or three days we felt it would never make it, so we stopped. And once we took a baby off the ventilator, we did not put it back because we felt that we had given the baby every opportunity to survive. If we had kept these babies on, we felt we would have created terrible damage. We didn't realize all the complications.

"Over a period of years all these things changed. We were able to dial in an exact amount of oxygen; we were able to measure the oxygen flow; we adapted the ventilator to babies, and we were able to ventilate smaller and smaller babies."

One turning point came when Dr. George Gregory and colleagues at the University of California developed CPAP (continuous positive airway pressure) ventilation. It allowed intubated babies to breathe out under pressure, so their frail lungs would never collapse completely. This was a big advance toward solving a major problem: the inability of premature lungs to stay open. The Baby Bird Ventilator, developed by Dr. Robert DeLemos, refined the technique even further, allowing a prolonging of inspiration, a constant flow as well as end-expiratory pressure. Work continued on ventilators, with large medical technology firms stepping in, so that in the decades to follow something new was always being tried out in the major research centers' nurseries.

The next major breakthrough, after ventilation, was in nutrition. Surgeons at the University of Pennsylvania, working with fetal puppies, developed a technique for providing nutrition intravenously to infants who could not absorb nourishment through their gastric systems. Hyperalimentation, or total parenteral nutrition (TPN), was designed to provide an infant's complete nutritional requirements in a mix that is infused through a catheter surgically implanted into the superior vena cava, one of the major blood vessels leading to the heart. It supplies a steady flow of amino acids, fats, proteins, carbohydrates, trace minerals, and other nutrients.

TPN was as great an advance in neonatology as ventilation, and it could similarly become a trap. Just as some infants became ventilator-dependent, surviving for a long time without ever being able to get off the machine, so a small proportion became permanently dependent on hyperalimentation. Their gastric systems never took over, and eventually they either had to be consciously disconnected from the life-support catheter or they died a slow and painful death.

As the research centers and the associated intensive care nurseries proliferated, the nation's infant mortality rate began to drop steadily. In 1974 it had halved, at 12.3. It continued its decline in the ensuing years by an average of 4.6 percent a year until 1982, almost entirely because fetuses that used to miscarry or die at birth were being saved in the ICNs, with the help of the new technology.

By the mid-1980s, neonatology was one of the fastest-growing areas in American medicine, and probably the fastest-growing field in pediatrics, according to Dr. Sunshine. "I'm basing this statement on several things: a third of the abstracts in research submitted to the national meetings of the American Pediatrics Society and the Society for Pediatric Research are related to the newborn or preemie. A third of the people going into postdoctoral training go into neonatology." The profitability of intensive care for hospitals, and a surplus of neonatologists who wanted to practice what they had learned, continued to feed the proliferation of ICNs, and competition for patients.

The most highly equipped nurseries, designated Level III or tertiary care centers, treated infants flown in or transported by ambulance from hospitals lacking the full array of medical specialists and life-support technology—designated Levels II and I, or intermediate and primary care centers. Whenever possible, pregnant women at high risk were brought to the advanced care hospital to deliver, for good results often depended on starting the babies' treatment before, during, or immediately after their birth.

As the research data mounted, the techniques for sustaining frail babies were refined and reports showing an improving outcome were published in journals. Respiratory distress syndrome was no longer commonly fatal. In the context of a modern ICN, three-pound babies were large. Neonatology continued to push back the threshold of viability.

But as the new interventions saved many lives and prevented disabilities in many infants, they also created a new population of disabled survivors. It was discovered that about 40 percent of the very low-birth-weight preterm babies, those weighing 1500 grams or less, had intraventricular brain hemorrhages of varied severity, putting them at risk for retardation, cerebral palsy, and other handicaps.[5] Most of those who remained on ventilators for more than two weeks developed chronic lung disease (CLD) or bronchopulmonary dysplasia (BPD). Their lung tissue became scarred, impeding the passage of air and interfering with the exchange of oxygen and carbon dioxide. The long-term prospects for such infants remained uncertain. It would take years and much research to learn their fate, and most follow-up efforts did not extend beyond three years.

In a report published in 1985, "Preventing Low Birthweight," an interdisciplinary committee of the Institute of Medicine, National Academy of Sciences, called attention to the fact that no national data system was being planned to look systematically at the relationship between low birth weight and subsequent morbidity.[6] The continuing growth of neonatology did not depend on long-term results. It was fueled in part by a surplus of neonatologists, in part by the profitability of intensive care nurseries to hospitals.

Meanwhile, innovations and advances in obstetrics and perinatology had also proceeded rapidly, feeding both progress and problems in neonatology. Pediatrics teams were installed in the delivery rooms of the most advanced hospitals, ready to support a baby if there was trouble. Techniques were developed for recognizing high-risk pregnancies, for monitoring diabetic women, for delaying the onset of labor, for monitoring the fetal heartbeat, and for estimating whether a baby's lungs were mature enough to allow survival after a premature birth. All these innovations meant an improved chance of health and well-being for many infants. They also meant that fetuses that would have ended as miscarriages grew to be viable babies. Combining with the interventions in the ICNs, these obstetrical advances added to the numbers of preterm infants who survived.

Technological expansion also brought new methods for detecting defects in fetuses, allowing parents to choose abortion instead of the birth of a seriously damaged child. Amniocentesis, a procedure usually performed between the sixteenth and eighteenth weeks of gestation, can yield information on more than fifty chromosomal and inherited biochemical abnormalities, particularly Down's syndrome. It involves removing a sample of the amniotic fluid that surrounds a fetus by inserting a hollow needle in the mother's abdomen. In the late 1970s, many obstetricians were recommending the procedure for all women over age thirty-five, because older women are at higher risk for delivering Down's syndrome babies.

The maternal serum alpha-fetoprotein (AFP) test is effective in detecting almost all cases of anencephaly, the absence of all or a major part of the brain, and two-thirds of the cases of spina bifida. The amniotic fluid is analyzed for the presence of excessive levels of alpha-fetoprotein, a substance that is manufactured by the fetal liver in the first fifteen weeks of gestation and normally excreted through the urine. Excessive amounts of AFP in the fluid after the fifteenth week indicate the possibility of faulty development that has left an open spinal column. The results of this test are verified by ultrasound and sometimes by amniocentesis as well.

Ultrasound scanning, which was originally developed for military purposes to detect the presence of ships and submarines, is used to create a picture of the fetus that shows size, position and formation, its age and condition, and reveals some defects. The sonar scanner bounces a beam of sound waves off the internal structures of mother and fetus. It can pick up a heartbeat and movement and has been found so useful that in Germany, women routinely undergo two scans during pregnancy.[7] The procedure has been used far less widely in the United States.

Another, more recent prenatal diagnostic technique is chorionic villi sampling, which has the advantage of being possible in the first trimester of pregnancy. Guided by ultrasound, a very thin plastic catheter is inserted through the vagina and cervix into the chorion, a layer of tissue that develops into the placenta. A sample is taken from the villi, tiny projections from the chorion, which transfer oxygen, nutrients, and wastes between mother and embryo. The procedure allows detection of Down's syndrome and chromosomal abnormalities. It is viewed as a possible alternative to amniocentesis. However, there is a risk of miscarriage, the magnitude of which has not yet been established.

The availability of prenatal diagnostic tests that yield results only late in the pregnancy has created new dilemmas: fetuses are being aborted at an age when they are possibly candidates for survival as preemies. The convergence of these varied technological and medical developments in obstetrics and neonatology, therefore, has raised unprecedented ethical questions for everyone involved. In some hospitals, physicians and nurses have refused to perform abortions on fetuses older than twenty-two weeks, having seen babies of almost that gestational age being sustained with life-support equipment in the nursery. "I myself have not resolved this dichotomy," said Dr. Sunshine. "It is the biggest problem that I see right now."

The dilemma is, at least in part, a consequence of the direction that medicine has taken—toward intensive care rather than, as would have been possible, toward public health measures that would have prevented some of the damage that the high-tech nurseries try to repair. That prevention was neglected is starkly clear. In 1985, while high-risk nurseries were expanding and the national cost of newborn intensive care grew beyond $2 billion a year, there was a reported shrinkage in the proportion of women who received adequate prenatal care. Public spending on preventive health care and social programs was being curtailed.

By 1985 the point of diminishing returns had been reached in many ways. The rate of improvement in the infant mortality rate dropped to half of what it had been and, according to the United States Public Health Service, seemed to be stabilizing at about eleven per thousand. Despite the improvements in the preceding decades, the nation had continued to slip in its ranking among industrialized nations. It stood in seventeenth place in 1982, while Finland and Japan were the leaders, with Sweden close behind. The goal of nine per thousand that the surgeon general had set in 1979 for 1990 was receding.[8] In addition, a slight rise was noted in the postneonatal mortality rate (deaths of infants aged twenty-eight days to twelve months). Although such deaths have been correlated with poverty, lack of sanitation, and similar socioeconomic factors, there was reason to believe that a number were related to intensive care: some babies were not saved; their death was merely postponed.

Improvements continued to be made in intensive care of premature infants, but a threshold seemed to have been reached. Neonatologists were looking at a biological limit. Infants younger than twenty-five or so weeks' gestation and smaller than 500 grams (1 lb. 2 oz.) did not, with rare exceptions, survive in the ICNs. They were too immature to be supported by the existing technology.

The dramatic progress in the high-risk nurseries had masked, but not affected, the major contributor to infant mortality, prematurity. Voices began to call for a look in a different direction. In February 1985, the Committee to Study the Prevention of Low Birthweight urged that a national commitment be made to ensure that all pregnant women receive high-quality prenatal care. "The overwhelming weight of the evidence" shows that "prenatal care reduces the risk of low birthweight," the group stated.[9]

Perinatologists say they do not know what triggers labor and that insufficient scientific evidence exists on why some women go into labor early. Considerable data does exist, however, on who is at risk for giving birth early: teenagers, smokers, women who go through severe emotional stress, women who have had various infections, women who work at hard manual labor, women who are poor, and women who receive no prenatal care. Information is available on efforts that have successfully reduced prematurity, at a cost way below that of keeping frail newborns alive, though this information may not stand up to strict scientific examination. Therefore, for those who believe that society's efforts would have been better spent on prevention, what was "apparent" was not "the need for" premature research centers and ICNs, as the Stanford Premature Infant Research Center people saw it, but much greater effort to assure adequate prenatal care and support for all pregnant women.

Neonatologists at Stanford agree that prevention is by far the better option. Their major responsibility, however, is the babies they save, and their families. By 1985 the big issue in neonatal units was not mortality but morbidity. The challenge was to ensure that the tiny rescued babies would grow into normal, healthy people.

Neonatology began to move into the basic sciences—biology, biochemistry, physiology. Some of the most promising work was being done in molecular physiology. Techniques were developed to monitor metabolic processes without disturbing infants and to gather information about potential problems before they escalated into illness. One of the most promising among these is trace gas analysis, the study of exhaled gases, which allows the monitoring of digestive and other metabolic processes.

Several institutions now monitor hydrogen gas, which is produced by bacteria as they ferment carbohydrates in the intestine. If improperly absorbed in the small intestine, carbohydrates reach the large intestine and ferment there. The presence of an excessive amount of hydrogen in a baby's breath signals malabsorption of carbohydrates or sugar intolerance.

The breath carries more than two hundred other constituents, so if they can be detected and their sources traced, an enormous new window will open into the functioning of the metabolism in a living person. Already, neonatologists have begun to learn about basic physiology through this technique. They have observed, for instance, that premature infants do not, like older humans, absorb most of their carbohydrates in the small intestine. Some of the absorption takes place in the large intestine, with the help of bacteria, as happens in such ruminants as cows.

At Stanford, research has also begun on exhaled carbon monoxide as an indicator of the risk of jaundice. This gas is produced, along with bilirubin, or jaundice pigment, as hemoglobin breaks down. It is excreted in parts per million in the baby's breath. By measuring it in the breath, one can estimate the production rate of bilirubin. The procedure may provide an earlier warning signal than blood sampling does, and has the immense advantage of not disturbing the baby at all. Eventually, trace gas analysis may permit the study of a baby's response to various interventions on the molecular level.

Neonatology is on the cutting edge of medical science in the development of such refined monitoring technology because many tools used elsewhere in medical practice are too crude for the delicate beings in the ICN. The sampling of blood may not bother an adult much, but some of the extremely small babies have two ounces or less in their entire circulatory system, so losing 0.2 or 0.3 cc several times a day is no small matter. Besides being painful, the procedure necessitates frequent blood replacement by transfusion.

Eventually, some of the refinements achieved in neonatology are adopted more broadly, because they are more effective and less invasive than methods used previously. One example is the transcutaneous oxygen probe, which is sometimes an alternative to blood sampling. A sensor is placed on the skin, usually somewhere on the trunk. It warms the tissue and allows the measurement of carbon dioxide and oxygen as they diffuse from the blood and through the skin to the sensor.

The move toward molecular medicine is leading toward possible development of antiviral agents, of drugs that will affect the growth of the lungs and the maturing of the gastrointestinal system. It does not exclude innovations along more conventional lines, of course. Experiments have begun at several centers in extracorporeal circulation, the use of modified heart/lung machines to replenish oxygen in the infant's blood outside the body, bypassing the lungs. The hope is to avoid ventilator-caused damage, but as usual, the new technique is sure to bring a new set of hazards. As has been true many times before, in the time of Dr. Budin's "child hatchery," during the first experiments with ventilators and in other risky research, moribund babies are being used as subjects of heart/lung machine experiments.

Organ transplants are a likely development for the future. At Stanford, the policy in 1985 was that not enough data existed to support such measures with infants. They were not, of course, ruled out for later. The artificial placenta may be feasible, but is probably "two or three major advances down the line," one neonatologist said. The information about growth and development from the middle of the second trimester of gestation is still too scanty.

"Right now I don't see anything in the foreseeable future keeping babies much smaller alive," reflected Dr. Sunshine. Then he paused and added, "Although I said the same thing when we got down to 1000 grams."

The intensive care nursery at Stanford is a world unto itself. Though its windows can offer a glimpse of the world beyond, their pink and orange curtains are often drawn. Even when they are not, what goes on within is so compelling that, in a sense, the outside world ceases to exist. On any day or night, between twenty-five and forty infants lie enmeshed in the tentacles of life-support equipment, held in suspension at the threshold of life in the hope that they will rally enough strength to breathe, eat, and grow.

The Stanford University Medical Center is a warren of special worlds. Down the hall to the west, healthy full-term babies are delivered, taken into their mother's arms, and soon sent home, as are some 90 percent of all infants born in the United States.

In the pediatrics ward to the north, older children—some of whom were born at the center and saved in the ICN from dying—are being treated for various ailments, awaiting surgery, or recovering from it. Some have come from distant places, even from abroad. Parents with sad eyes sit at their bedsides.

Across another hall, to the south, languish adult cancer patients, hoping that, in this so-very-modern medical center, a cure might exist for their disease. Their visitors share the lounge with families of the newborn ICN patients. Farther to the south, in another wing of the building, medical students attend classes and study. In scattered laboratories, researchers bend over experiments that may soon make headlines. Deep down in the basement, microbiologists have been growing rat brain cells and performing surgery on them in hopes of learning more about the human brain, architect of all that goes on here.

The people who come to this medical center are diverse. Among the 23,000 admitted annually to the 663 bed hospital, and those making 140,000 visits to the outpatient clinics, are some who can afford the best that money can buy and some so poor that bus fare is a serious item in the budget. They include many Hispanic and Asian immigrants as well as native Americans who are as varied ethnically as the people of California. Many have been referred from outlying hospitals because their problems are too rare or difficult for institutions that lack the full array of technology and expertise.

The Stanford Medical School, with some four hundred students, prides itself in training not only doctors but future leaders of the profession. There is a heavy emphasis on research, and many graduates aspire to academic medicine. Major research interests include a center for molecular and genetic medicine.

Since the fifty-six-acre, $27 million complex was built in 1959, it has been at the forefront of medical technology. The first six-million-volt linear accelerator for cancer treatment in the Western Hemisphere was installed here in 1956. The first North American heart transplant was achieved in 1968 by Dr. Norman E. Shumway, to be followed by 350 more by 1985, a fourth of the transplants worldwide.

Other pioneering work includes development of lasers to weld on detached retinas and the first reported extensive electrical simulations of the auditory nerve in man to treat deafness. In the 1960s, Drs. Henry S. Kaplan and Saul Rosenberg, researchers, developed a combination of drug and radiation treatment for Hodgkin's disease, which until then had almost always been fatal.

As the reputation of the medical center has grown, fueled by research funds (grants from the National Institutes of Health in 1983–1984 totaled $66 million) so have space requirements. By 1985 a new wing was under construction, necessitating the destruction of part of an addition that was only six years old. It was to include a new and more spacious intensive care nursery. Meanwhile, the existing nursery, opened twenty-five years earlier and remodeled in 1981, in many ways reflected the state of the art of intensive care for very sick or very small newborns.

The ICN is a long, bright room, lit night and day with the same white intensity. It could be a space-age laboratory. Along its length has been deployed a vast array of hardware laden with switches, dials, and digital clocks. Plugged into the walls are machines that pump, pulse, suction, and calibrate. Electronic monitors continually trace waves and spikes on video screens, spew out patterned paper ribbons, emit flashing signals that occasionally beep in alarm. Men and women in pastel cotton suits or gowns move about, watching the oscillation of hundreds of needles, adjusting knobs, writing on flow charts attached to clipboards, wheeling around still more gadgetry that photographs and scans. The ambient sound is of muffled voices against a background of steady mechanical hiss, punctuated by bleeps and screeches. This is the place to which babies are rushed from the delivery room when the natural birth process has gone amiss and medical science steps in to make amends.

The babies lie in two rows parallel to the windows, in the rectangular transparent plastic isolettes, in bassinets or cribs, or on slanted hotbeds—platforms set under radiant lamps. Some of them are so small and scrawny that they really are more fetus than baby. The tiniest have arms no thicker than an adult's finger, heels as small as the eraser at the end of a pencil. The blood volume of each one totals about six tablespoons. Mostly naked, they lie froglike on their bellies and splayed on their backs or curled—as they should surely have remained in their mothers' wombs—attached by tubes and wires and needles to the surrounding equipment.

The uninitiated entering the place for the first time are shocked, remembering college zoology laboratories. Some of the babies have huge sutures. Some are dark red or bluish. Most appear immobile. It is not immediately clear that they are alive. Occasionally there is the sound of an infant cry, which makes the place even more eerie, for it calls attention to the fact that most of these infants make no sound at all. The first-time visitor to the intensive care nursery often recoils in confusion and fear.

A Mexican-American farmworker who saw his baby here bowed his head, made the sign of the cross, and then told the social worker, "I have no money for the funeral." But his baby was not dead, only paralyzed as part of the therapy. Some months later, the family sent a snapshot of a chubby-cheeked infant with a note expressing gratitude to the nursery staff.

The vast majority of the approximately one thousand infants who pass through the Stanford ICN every year go home and grow up to be normal. That is hard to believe as one first looks at these pitiful patients. About 20 percent of the high-risk infants continue to have significant problems.

The infant patients can be grouped into four categories: those who are being observed because of the mother's history or an event during the delivery; those with congenital birth defects that might be corrected by surgery; those who are acutely ill; and those who are born too soon to adjust to the environment outside the womb without technical assistance. A small fifth group are infants who are born dying and cannot be aided by doctors' knowledge and skills—fetuses that remain alive after a miscarriage or abortion just prior to the age of viability and babies lacking most of the brain. They are brought here to be made as comfortable as possible until they expire or, in some cases, are sent home to die.

The first group, babies under observation, includes infants of diabetic mothers, who are at risk for congenital heart disease and other malformations and whose blood sugar must be monitored in the first days; infants of women who, during pregnancy, took medications that are known to be harmful to a fetus: tranquilizers, sedatives, anticonvulsants, steroids, and other substances. Another group in the first category includes infants born to women with active hepatitis and herpes and to addicts of alcohol or narcotics. The addicts' babies are born physically addicted and must be helped through withdrawal.

Also in this category are babies who were injured during delivery or asphyxiated at birth, perhaps because the umbilical cord was wrapped around their neck, and some who stayed too long in the womb—over forty-two weeks instead of the thirty-eight to forty that is the normal gestational age—and are at risk because they may be malnourished, asphyxiated, and may have inhaled some meconium-stained amniotic fluid. Meconium, a normal greenish-black sticky material in the fetal intestine, is usually excreted during the first days after birth but is sometimes released in the uterus when the fetus is in distress. If a baby inhales it, serious respiratory and other problems can occur.

Among the second category, birth-defect babies, are some with abnormalities that, under current conditions, can be easily repaired by a competent surgeon. But there are also some whose visible defects signal further abnormalities that are far more difficult to evaluate—the spina bifida infants, for instance.

Babies acutely ill with infections—viral, bacterial, respiratory, septic—require the full array of interventions available, but they may soon recover and please their families and doctors by growing up healthy and normal.

A senior pediatrics resident, who plans to be a neonatologist, says his greatest satisfaction has come from babies in the acutely ill group. He remembers a boy who had aspirated meconium and had severe pneumonia and abnormal pulmonary circulation. "Kids like that—you use maximum support, the kind a preemie could never stand. They're our sickest kids and they get better and they're normal. You burn out two or three house officers when you get a kid like that. You sit there at the bedside for hours. They're hard to manage. You change one little thing and it sends them spiraling. But they're mostly home in a month. They're worth the fight. The others, I don't know; there's some question there for me."

These others are in the fourth category in the nursery, preterm low-birth-weight (LBW) infants. This group accounts for most of neonatology's spectacular successes, and to many is the most troubling ethically.

The World Health Organization has defined an LBW infant as one weighing less than 2500 grams (5½ lb.) and a preterm infant as one born after less than thirty-seven weeks' gestation. The distinction is important because some 15 percent of the infants who weigh under five pounds at birth are term babies. They are called SGA—small for gestational age. Babies born at 1500 grams or less are customarily classified as VLBW, very low birth weight.

Infants who arrive after the twenty-eighth or twenty-ninth week and weigh in at two pounds or more usually do well in the ICN, even though many of them would have died only a few years ago. But the extremely small ones, the ones who weigh no more than 800 grams (1 lb. 12 oz.), and who were born early in the third trimester of pregnancy, face a treacherous course. Some become legendary "miracle babies," breathing on their own, beginning to grow, and going home at about the time they had been due to be born. But others linger, become chronically ill, suffer one mishap and setback after another, and eventually either die or leave at risk for a variety of handicaps.

The babies of less than 800 grams birth weight represent only 2 percent of the annual ICN population. Only half the babies this small make it out of the delivery room, and, of those who do, only half survive. If they become ill, they are at extremely high risk for death or disability. But little is known, overall, about their prospects. Only since 1982 have enough of them survived to permit any kind of statistical data gathering. They raise questions that make neonatologists uneasy. Dr. Ronald Ariagno puts it this way: "The purpose of all this technology is to heal. If whole normal infants do not result, what is the sense of it all?"

At forty-three, Dr. Ariagno had already been one of the three senior neonatologists at Stanford for ten years. He is a man of deep social conscience, powerful empathy, with a brilliant analytic mind, a capacity for total attention, and that essential survival gift, a sense of humor. He enjoys his staff's respect and affection. Some parents find him too blunt when he tells them bad news, but most appreciate his directness. He looks things straight in the eye and calls them by their names. He listens and worries about the consequences of what he is doing. Knowing that a high percentage of the premature infants whose lives are saved with respirators go home with chronic lung disease, he feels it urgent to press on with research to improve the outcome.

In many ways, Ron Ariagno is a man of his time and the kind of doctor who inspires others. He loves the space age and dreams of taking a sabbatical at NASA to research the possibilities for birth in space. He believes that human beings are incredibly resilient and astonishing, and that it would be wrong not to try to beat back death whenever an infant has a good chance of recovery.

But regarding the tiniest of newborns—the babies who are barely more than fetuses—he says, "We are all asking ourselves, Is it appropriate to be heroic? For some of the most immature infants, we need a placental unit rather than the other tools we now use in the ICN to obtain better results." He does not recommend, however, that an artificial womb be attempted, at least not right now. There are already enough unresolved ethical issues with the preemies without inviting more.

Very early preemies need incredible amounts of support: help with breathing, feeding, maintaining body temperature. They lack the baby fat that grows during the last trimester of gestation and allows adjustment to a changed environmental temperature. They also lack the energy reserves for other major physiological changes that occur dramatically and naturally in full-term infants at birth. Their entire system is too frail for the enormous stresses they must survive. They quickly use up such energy as they have and become vulnerable to various disorders and infections. Their capillaries leak easily, flooding the brain, injuring the eyes and the lungs. Their gastrointestinal system is often unready for the work it has to do later, so they must be fed intravenously. The treatment that keeps them alive often injures them and can cause permanent damage.

The major threshold they must pass is the transition to independent breathing. In the baby born in its time, the first breath, the first cry, triggers enormous changes in the lungs and the heart. Until that moment, oxygen has come through the placenta. Blood circulated through the body and flowed out into the placenta again, where it shed waste carbon dioxide and was once more replenished with oxygen. A fetal artery called the ductus arteriosus allowed most of the flow to bypass the lungs, which were still developing and filled with fluid.

Normally, labor prepares the baby to start breathing. The mother's contractions squeeze and massage the infant chest, helping to expel fluid from the lungs and stimulating the motions of breathing. As the baby emerges, air rushes in with the first breath, filling the alveoli, the tiny air sacs in the lungs. The blood vessels of the lungs expand and suddenly become the route of least resistance for the blood. A coating, called a surfactant, appears in the lungs, preventing their total collapse during exhalation, so that the next breath comes easily.

The heart adapts to the new circulation pattern. It is separated into two chambers when a flap of tissue in the atrium drops. Blood that has been oxygenated in the lungs flows into the left atrium and to the left ventricle. It is pumped from there through the body, returning to the right atrium and to the right ventricle laden with carbon dioxide. It then returns to the lungs, where it gets rid of the waste gas and fills with oxygen. The ductus arteriosus closes.

That is the pattern in a healthy baby born at term. But premature infants are not yet ready for this awesome process. For them the stresses that would later have been beneficial are harsh and dangerous. Contractions may asphyxiate these babies. The alveoli, lacking the surfactant, tend to collapse during exhalation and are then held shut by surface tension. Each breath becomes harder, and these tiny beings are soon exhausted by their effort.

The failure of the lungs to stay expanded allows the carbon dioxide–laden blood to continue flowing through the fetal ductus arteriosus and from there through the baby's body. This means that the infant gets too little oxygen—he gasps, his chest heaves and retracts, the heart beats too fast. The infant can succumb at this point to respiratory distress syndrome, a common major problem among very small preterm babies. Until the 1960s, when the respirator began to be used with such babies, little could be done about it, and RDS was the most common cause of death among premature infants. Now many survive, but a newborn who has to stay on the respirator for more than two weeks is highly likely to develop chronic lung disease, which he may or may not outgrow. His rate of recovery must outpace the damage that the respirator inflicts on his delicate lung tissues.

According to Dr. Ariagno, 67 percent of such infants—ventilated for two weeks and unable to be weaned—whose birth weight was under 1500 grams develop chronic lung disease. The smaller the baby, the higher the risk. Many outgrow the damage; up to 30 percent die, one-third after leaving the hospital.

In the ICN—as in much of modern medicine—therapy is always close to research and experimentation. Doctors sometimes say that each baby is its own experiment. This could perhaps be said of any critically ill patient, but it is especially true here because the technology is so new, the outcome data often nonexistent, and the patients so fragile. A tiny move can push them over the edge. "We are never totally in control of the dilemmas that evolve here," said Dr. Ariagno.

The neonatologists who direct the ICN, and who rotate monthly as attending physicians, are assisted by postgraduate neonatology fellows, pediatric residents and interns, and by a cadre of diverse specialists—respiratory and physical therapists, sonographers (who work with ultrasound), pharmacologists, radiologists, X-ray technicians, nutritionists, audiologists, ophthalmologists, consulting birth-defect specialists, cardiologists, neurosurgeons. Babies who are primarily surgical patients are the surgeons' responsibility, the rest the neonatologists'. Some babies are supervised by private doctors who are not on the staff but come to see them and confer with house physicians. All are cared for daily by special nurses who are assigned one to two small patients, depending on the intensity of treatment being provided.

A sense of intermittent emergency prevails as various babies become subject to the interventions of these groups of professionals who come and go alone or in teams. The bleeping alarm signals, which are false warnings much of the time, merely annoy the nurses. But they also announce genuine crises—a baby gasping for air, a tiny heart speeding up or slowing down. Then teams of practitioners swarm to intercede to keep a flickering life from expiring.

The diverse teams cooperate, but they also often disagree, for each brings its own particular perspective to bear. The result is an atmosphere of creative tension that is conducive to research and learning and can provide the most carefully reasoned and informed medical approach to treatment. It does not necessarily provide the continuity and tranquillity, however, that is needed for the nurture of delicate newborns.

The lights, never dimmed, are so bright that they may contribute to retinopathy of prematurity, a condition that historically has been associated with the administration of supplemental oxygen.[10] The acoustical environment is incessantly noisy. A study in two Southern California ICNs found that high-intensity and low-frequency sounds at potentially hazardous levels prevailed for extended periods. The authors found noise level "comparable to automobile traffic," and wrote that "at times the noise reached levels of large machinery." The same was true within incubators where, in addition, infants were subjected to continuous white noise generated by the isolette.[11]

The ICN environment conforms to the demands of the technology that made intensive care possible. It is alien to almost all who first enter it. It is especially alien to most parents.

The parents come at all hours. They are welcome at any time. At first there is only one real place for them in the bright room: the specific location where their own infant is installed and plugged in. In time, however, be it after a few hours or a few days, they begin to adapt, to see more, and finally to accept what at first seemed bizarre.

Privacy is absent. Parents who want to coo or sing to their baby must do so under the eyes of strangers. A few feet away are other infants, their nurses, other parents. While the parents of one may be sweet-talking their baby, another child may be struggling for breath. Nearby, another may be dying.

The lack of privacy is also a benefit, however, because it brings parents closer to each other and to the staff. The particular pain that parents of very premature or disabled infants suffer tends to separate them from relatives and friends, for it is outside the experience of all but a few. On viewing Polaroid snapshots of infants who look more like fetuses trapped within an experiment, most people don't know what to say. Congratulations do not seem to be in order, but neither are condolences. A secretary in one father's office, on seeing a 550 gram infant's picture, exclaimed, "How bizarre!" Others are more discreet, but often suppress a similar reaction. There is a human tendency to recoil from life forms that appear unnatural.

However, a full-term healthy newborn would be out of place among the preemies in the ICN. In this area, a seven- or eight-pounder looks too big. What starts out being shocking and strange gradually becomes the standard by which one imperceptibly measures.

The parent of a tiny premature infant cannot accept the advice of mothers of healthy term babies. For one thing, the ancient formula of holding and cuddling is contraindicated: premature infants are touched and disturbed as little as possible in the beginning. This seems to go against nature, as do many rules one learns in the ICN. So parents are relieved to see others who share their predicament.

Parents whose babies are in the ICN for a long time gradually get to know doctors and nurses as lifelines to their children. And, as the weeks stretch into months and the daily visits to the hospital continue, the entire ICN becomes central to many parents' lives. They have little time for other social activities, and the intensity of their concern and involvement with the hospital builds higher the wall that began to rise when they first showed around their odd baby pictures.

Like any community, the ICN has its own politics, customs, and language. As time goes on, many parents begin to assume them and slip into new speech patterns speckled with freshly learned terms: CMV, PDA, CPAP, RDS. The numbers on the dials of the life-support equipment become the gauge of their infant's well-being. "His settings were lower today and his O's were really good," some will say in response to a question about how the baby is doing. Drawn into this intense separate world, they become a part of it. Their friends and associates must bear with them until their baby comes home.

In the entryway of the nursery is a bulletin board on which are posted many snapshots of healthy ICN graduates, plump babies and small children who look reassuringly fine. There are letters of gratitude from parents, among them one that ends, "You saved his life and gave him the chances he needed in his struggle for survival. The horrible two months he spent with wires, tubes, and monitors attached to his little body are only hazy memories."

CHAPTER THREE

The ICN as a Separate Culture

Dr. Molly Summers's long blond hair hangs loose around a rosy plump face. She is a friendly, warm young woman, and it is hard to think of her as a doctor, unless you watch her at work. She sat in the cafeteria, in slacks and heavy wool turtleneck sweater, tired and feeling immensely relieved. She had survived her first month's rotation as an intern in the intensive care nursery—a month that was, by everyone's measure, horrendous. Twice the usual number of babies had died in the unit and more than the usual number had gone home with rare and severe birth defects. The entire staff was emotionally exhausted and had aired a lot of grievances during the last nursery management meeting. The attending physician took the brunt of nurses' criticism. But it had been a hard month for him no less. Sometimes, as he looked at a baby, the image of the one who had been in that particular spot just hours earlier—the one he had tried to save and couldn't— would flash before his mind.

Three of the minute ones who died had been Dr. Summers's responsibility. The two interns and one junior resident on a team divide the nursery into three parts, each taking responsibility for about ten infants. They work as peers, overseen by the senior resident who answers to the fellow and the attending physician. Molly Summers had spent hours with the fetus who had died two nights before, whose mother was in her thirties and had two other children, and whose father was only sixteen years old. And she had worked all night on the other tiny one, who had died in the morning.

Late one afternoon, she had walked into the conference room and found Charlene Canger, the social worker, with some parents, looking at a film about babies dying. She had started to cry and could not stop.

Before this month, Dr. Summers had never even set foot in the ICN. Looking back, she recalled that her first reaction was "fear and something similar to—I hate to use the word *disgust*, but I felt almost offended by some of the things that, not knowing, I thought could not possibly be right to do to a child. Just looking at some of the kids strapped down, all their extremities pinned down, lines going up, IVs in their heads and in their hands, becoming blue and edematous from the paralyzing, with no stimulation except lights and noise—to me it was awful. In some ways I still think it is, but you kind of get used to it."

Having broken down so uncontrollably, she had gone to see the attending, to ask him, "What about these babies' future, and what about the pain they must be experiencing?" The answers she received failed to satisfy her. She was troubled, not just about what she had to do to the babies, but also about what she felt was happening to her.

"I recognized the babies as humans and felt for them, but not as much as I would have liked to have felt. There is a certain very significant degree of turning off your feelings—just as a defense mechanism, because otherwise you would be falling apart. I found myself really pulling away from the kids and just looking at their numbers and their weights and their inputs and their outputs and their electrolytes and all that stuff, not really looking at them, at their faces, and not touching them that much—in order not to feel sad about the state they are in.

"These babies—sometimes it's just like a room full of objects, all lined up in a row, all plugged in. Many times I felt so horrible, because I felt I was contributing to their suffering." She knew that others distanced themselves from the pain in many ways. But she also thought that, perhaps, others did not feel what she felt quite so much.

"From what I can tell, the further up you get in your studying here, the more cold you get, the more distant. I think that is inevitable, but I don't think it's necessary and I don't think it's good. I think it's bad and it's scary that it would happen to me."

The young doctors who endure the enormously stressful ICN service sometimes speak of being "on the front lines" or "in the trenches." And indeed, one way to view the nursery is as a war zone, where special forces and armaments are deployed against death and disability. As in war or other intense, separate, and dangerous contexts—mountain-climbing expeditions, natural disasters, storms at sea—survival and well-being in the ICN demand teamwork. People come to know one another well, they help one another in crises, they hold together against the rest of the world, knowing that nobody who has not shared their experience can fully understand. They develop their own special ways of seeing and doing things, their own special language and humor. In effect, they become a separate small society. Another way to look at the ICN is as a micro-society, with its unique culture.

Eugene B. Brody, a psychiatrist, and Howard Klein, a pediatrician and family practitioner at the University of Maryland School of Medicine, presented such a description in an article published in the British journal *Paediatrician* in September 1980. They point out that the ICN has many characteristics of a small society. Though unique, it also mirrors the society of which it is a part, reflecting value problems arising with a rapid advance of technology. As portrayed by Brody and Klein, the ICN society has two discrete and incongruous aspects: the technological, which separates and dehumanizes, and the caring, which tries to nurture and heal.

The diverse adults who busy themselves with the babies in the ICN can be broadly divided into two subcultures, with different values and social structures: the physicians and their various technical assistants, and the nurses and social support staff. The first is focused primarily on treatment and saving life, research and teaching; the second is concerned with caring, alleviation of suffering, and nurture of relationships. The first is goal-oriented, the second process-oriented. The first is organized in a strictly hierarchical manner; the second shares responsibility in a more horizontal pattern. As the two groups must and do work together, the complementarity between them becomes evident. A major reason given by staff members, both physicians and nurses, for liking this particular nursery was that the nurses are strong and independent, working with rather than for the doctors. But the first group is dominant.

Though there are men among the nurses and a sizable proportion of the interns and residents are women, the physician group is dominated by men; the other is composed primarily of women, as is typical throughout American medicine. Ethicist John Golenski, a Jesuit priest and administrator at Children's Hospital Medical Center in Oakland, California, has observed that the different values of the two ICN staff groups reflect gender-linked value differences that have recently come to the attention of social researchers.

Studies by William Perry, Lawrence Kohlberg, and Carol Gilligan at Harvard have shown that men and women tend to follow different paths in their moral development and arrive at different sets of values. According to Gilligan, men progress toward a morality of rights and an understanding of fairness; women grow toward recognition of differences in need, relationship, and responsibility.[1]

In the ICN, both a dichotomy and a complementarity can be seen in interactions between the physician teams and the nursing and social support teams. Golenski sees the value differences expressed in the way the two groups relate to the infants: "How often have I heard a neonatologist say, 'I have to give that kid a chance to live. I have to give him an opportunity. The baby will decide for us.' A nurse, on the other hand, is more likely to say, 'I cannot stand to see this pain any longer. I cannot, in light of my own integrity, continue to inflict pain, deny this baby the dignity of a human being in the process of dying.'"

A sense of fairness and individual rights is pitted against a sense of relationship and compassion. The goal-oriented battle for life is tempered by attention to the existence of suffering. The physicians, wielding technology and drawing on their therapeutic skills and techniques, are the strategic arms command and the generals in the war against death. The nurses are Berthold Brecht's Mother Courage—bandaging wounds, ladling out food to the weary, even as they lament the cruelty of the total predicament. But the war metaphor is the doctors'. Nurses seldom speak in military terms about their work. The ICN is a creation of the dominant male value system. The steady, consistent presence of the nurses, however, exerts considerable power. The two groups together run the ICN society.

Decision making is collaborative. Nurses are routinely present during conferences between physicians and parents. Regular nursery management meetings provide a formal opportunity for nurses to voice concerns and complaints. The nurses are outspoken, and Dr. Sunshine said the meetings have on occasion been "quite painful" to physicians. When withdrawal of aggressive support becomes an issue during an ethics committee meeting or within a smaller group, the protocol is to continue as long as one person in the group thinks that further discussion might be worthwhile. Most staff disagreements are worked out amicably. This is not always true when physicians come in from outside the ICN community.

Late one summer afternoon, two pediatricians and a neurosurgeon had a showdown at an infant's bedside over whose prerogative it was to tap the ventricular space within his brain. The neuro team walked in as a pediatrics resident was about to perform the procedure on a twenty-seven-weeker who badly needed relief from the pressure within his skull, a consequence of a cerebral hemorrhage. The resident had all his equipment spread out on a stool, beside the baby. The nurse had disconnected the monitoring equipment and placed the infant across the bed, head at the edge, the rest of him covered with a blue blanket. The resident was standing beside the baby and putting on his gloves when the appearance of the neurosurgery team checked him.

As usual, these consultants, on their own schedule, had arrived unexpectedly, without coordinating with the nursery staff. They had come to do the job for which the resident was preparing. The leader, a stocky man wearing a casually opened white coat, walked in like a warlord with his retinue, his face displaying a disdainful smile. Alongside and slightly behind him came a surgery intern, carrying a clipboard, and a surgery resident, wearing street clothes.

"You have something to tell me?" inquired the neurosurgeon, looking around at the pediatricians. "My experience is that when twelve pediatricians come at me, they have something to tell me."

Only three pediatricians were present—the resident about to do the tap, a neonatology fellow, and the attending physician, who had happened to stop by at that moment. But the atmosphere was charged.

The attending replied that he had nothing special to say, that he had just been finishing rounds. Then he moved away to take a phone call, leaving his fellow and resident to deal with the standoff that was shaping up. The leading neurosurgeon laid the gauntlet: "If we are to be a consult service, I have been specif-ically told by my attending that we should do all the taps."

The neonatology fellow tried to be reasonable, but there was an edge to his voice. "Look," he said, "this is a teaching hospital. We need practice in this procedure." Soon the resident would be out in the community, without support of the more experienced phy-sicians at the center.

The neurosurgeon replied that his attending had been clear in his view that taps were the surgeons' prerogative and responsi-bility. (The attending neonatologist later agreed that that was cor-rect. At times, though, he added, neurological consultants have taught and delegated the procedure to a senior pediatrician.)

The pediatrics resident said nothing, but he began to get red in the face. He had put on his gloves and was holding the needle, all the while glaring at the neurosurgeon. He continued to stand above the baby. The nurse was on the baby's other side, holding her hands soothingly on his feet. The doctors continued to argue over territorial rights to the baby's skull, the neurosurgeon asser-tively, like a trial lawyer, the pediatrician quietly. The fellow made a conciliatory move, suggesting that they all take turns at this. But the neurosurgeon gave no ground, repeating what he had said before, almost in identical words: that his attending had been very clear. Finally, the pediatrics resident put down the needle, stripped off his gloves, and stepped away.

The neurosurgeon took over and played his moment before his audience—his two companions, the watching pediatricians, the primary nurse, and a few other observers who were slightly far-ther away. "Peanut-sized skull," he observed, picking up the needle. "But no problem. This baby has garage-sized ventricles. No way to miss." He inserted the needle through the skin, then pulled the scalp slightly to one side and thrust farther. He held a test tube under the top end of the hollow needle. A few dark red drops fell into it, then there were no more.

"You see, you can't do it with a twenty-five-gauge needle; you need the twenty-two," he informed the pediatricians triumphantly.

"I've done several with the twenty-five," came the reply.

No more dark drops came. The neurosurgeon pulled out the needle. "That's why you need the twenty-two," he said, and he changed needles. Dark red filled the test tube. The color signaled that the insertion had been successful. Had the blood been bright red, it would have indicated that an artery had been punctured, something that can happen in this procedure. There is no way to see exactly where the needle is going. But statistically, the chances of benefit are greater than the chances of damage. Usually, the tap is done lower down, on the spine. But in this case a clot had developed, blocking flow of the bloody spinal fluid. The ventricular tap would be repeated several more times during the next two weeks until the baby's swollen head was down to appropriate size.

The neurosurgeon was explaining all this to the audience as the blood continued dripping into the test tube. He was clearly conscious of his stage presence. "That's how I used to get gas in 1973," he cracked, drawing a chuckle from his resident. At last the neurosurgeon pulled out the needle and held up the fluid-filled tube for a look. "Protein, glucose, and ozone rating. Why don't you write that down," he instructed his intern.

His resident laughed. "That would be good."

As the neurosurgery team withdrew, the nurse who had been holding the infant throughout the procedure bent toward him, her long hair making a curtain on both sides of his tiny head. "So many things they do to you," she said softly. She wiped his head with Betadine, soothing him with her hands. She reattached the electrodes, which had been removed for the duration of the tap, to continue to monitor his heart, respiration, and temperature. "It's all over now," she told the baby. "I'm done. That was awful, wasn't it?" Then she held him between the palms of her hands until he was quiet. The battle was over, the nurse tending the wounded.

The incident was a vivid illustration of the different ways doctors and nurses tend to relate to their tiny patients. For the physicians, what mattered was the procedure, its appropriate execution, territorial rights, and, in the case of the pediatricians, their need to learn how to do it. The nurse's attention, meanwhile, was focused on the infant's experience.

This incident also bore out Brody and Klein's observation that the most important members of this small society, the infants, are the least recognizably human, and can therefore be treated in ways that others would not be. Certainly even the least sensitive of physicians would acknowledge the presence of a conscious adult patient while inserting a needle into his head.

It is easy, however, under pressure of the duties at hand, for any physician to forget the fetus/baby as person—much easier for the physician, who has many patients, than for the nurse who has one or two. Sometimes it takes a conscious effort to see the extremely premature baby as more than an organism.

Physicians who choose pediatrics as a specialty are apt to be, as a group, of a gentler cast than, for instance, surgeons. They are, after all, people who like children. But their diminutive patients are far from being children or babies in the usual sense.

"In neonatology, babies don't respond much. They're organisms," said a senior pediatrics resident. "In a lot of ways it's like veterinary medicine. What you find in an exam is what the baby becomes, what a baby is: the baby with the murmur, the baby with congenital heart disease. Interaction with the baby is minimal. All you have is your history from someone else."

The pressures on their time, and the ICN environment, distance doctors from the little beings under their care. "We rely almost completely on the nurses," for information on what the babies might be feeling, said this resident. "They say things like 'This kid's off the wall.' Our job is to go from camp to camp putting out fires."

In their article, Brody and Klein postulated that new staff people coming to work in the ICN, particularly new house officers, "would undergo twin experiences of socialization and enculturation. They would learn the rules and habits of conformity in accordance with the power structure of the unit; and they would acquire some of the socially transmitted myths and beliefs about it."[2] They looked at the experience of interns, specifically, and concluded that the process of socialization they observed might have a deleterious impact on the infants.

The interns they studied went through a recognizable progression during their eight-week service in the nursery. They came with expectations, anticipating challenge. Once on service, they felt they had to demonstrate competence before they had quite overcome their bewilderment. They also felt a need to save face. They felt deprived of the human contact that patients in other hospital units provide. When they found they could not rescue babies for whom they were given responsibility, they were afflicted with guilt and shame. Then they questioned their work and wondered whether they should be doing it. They repressed their feelings, denied them, or became cynical. They performed painful interventions on children, shutting themselves off from compassion.

As the interns continued in the nursery, as they saw paradoxes, and as they became increasingly exhausted and angry, their feelings began to revolve around their relationships with other staff members. They tended to feel persecuted, to see nurses as adversaries, and to view residents with ambivalence.

At the end of their ICN service, interns felt that things fell into place. But afterwards, Brody and Klein observed a startling process: "Much of the experience is *sealed off*. The feeling of fright, helplessness, and hopelessness is forgotten and, by some, even denied. It is reminiscent of the sealing off which occurs after an acute psychotic episode when the patient resists going back and remembering what happened."[3] Most interns showed no interest in returning to the experience to make it better for their successors.

The authors of this study suggested that as these young physicians move up in the hierarchy, they are likely to punish other interns as they felt they themselves were punished. The small society's training of its leaders would thus be repeated without much change, with uncertain effects on the infants who serve as the teaching material, and on the future course of medicine.

The study was based on one nursery where the relationships between staff members were perhaps more fraught with conflict than is true at Stanford. But here, as in all other teaching hospitals, internship and residency are times when young doctors learn not only skills but also the attitudes, beliefs, and values of their profession.

Twice a day, at 8:00 A.M. and again at 3:00 P.M., someone places a sign, "Rounds in Progress," in the middle of the floor at the entrance to the nursery, and the medical team gathers at the nursery door for ward rounds. The attending physician, fellow, residents, and interns are usually accompanied by the charge nurse, a pharmacist, a social support team member, and occasionally by visiting medical professionals or researchers. The group—sometimes numbering as many as ten—proceeds bed by bed, stopping to talk about each baby.

Rounds are a transmission rite. They serve as briefing for the staff coming on duty, as a vehicle for teaching, and play a role in the enculturation of new members of the medical profession.

It is the task of the intern who was on call during the night to present the patients in the morning. This presentation is an op-portunity to demonstrate competence by giving a clear, concise report, asking some bright questions, showing one has made some intelligent decisions. The proper form is to describe the baby system by system—cardiovascular, digestive, respiratory, neuromuscular—with varied inflow and output occurring at dif-ferent speeds, intervals, pressures, and intensities. Nothing sig-nificant must be omitted, but there must be no lingering over nonessential detail. The intern strives for a tone that is authori-tative, snappy, and smooth during the recitation of the numbers he or she has collected. She may be bewildered, but she tries to give the impression she is at ease and knows what is going on. It is important to make the presentation with a certain panache.

That rounds are an occasion when socialization of young doc-tors occurs was evident one morning when it was Sam's turn. Sam was new and he was nervous. He was himself, as a persona, somewhat inappropriate. His presence spilled into the space around him rather than staying tight around a center. He was not particularly large physically, but he somehow took up more space than others did. As he gave his report, he kept pulling out a large gray handkerchief and wiping his forehead or blowing his nose. A resident remarked that he was lucky that Dr. Sunshine—who had strong ideas about nose blowing in the nursery—was not there, but Sam did not seem to hear. He didn't have a cold; it was a nervous tic, and he kept pulling out that rag—a cloth handker-chief, not a disposable tissue—as he moved along.

His way of giving the report was likewise inappropriate. Instead of looking around at the others or up and down at the flow sheet, he kept directing himself to a fellow intern, a soft-spoken young woman with long, shining brown hair. He even leaned toward her as he spoke.

He was not without wit; in fact he was extremely quick-minded, but when he tried—and even when he succeeded in—being funny, he was just a little too emphatic and too obvious in looking for a response. The other interns tossed off their lines "M*A*S*H"-style. Sam was definitely unsocialized, and he was becoming the subject of teasing that was faintly patronizing. Sometimes Sam stumbled over his numbers, sometimes he did not have them all, and once he waxed apologetic. "I was told it had been ordered." There was a note of complaint, of blame, in his voice—totally bad form. He had a lot to learn. But he did learn. By the end of the month, the teasing had become affectionate. "Sam, I'd be very careful on this baby," warned a resident. "You screw up on this one and you're in court."

"Why is that?"

"Parents are attorneys."

On one of his final days in the nursery, he was muttering the numbers with the speed and smoothness that matched anyone's, and he was also delivering his lines properly: "Johnson. Thirty weeks," 1800 grams. Kid acts irritable, becomes particularly irritable just before feedings, then gulps down 75 ccs, nippling, so it seems that the kid is [pause] hungry." He got a chuckle and did not spoil it by looking around for an effect.

Doctors sometimes talk among themselves in ways that might seem flip to people who do not have to face critically ill patients daily. Even to people who have watched "M*A*S*H," some of the ICN talk might be disconcerting.

"We see nothing but problems. They are alarming, even frightening," explained one of the senior physicians. "We don't have good solutions for them, so we act out a little bit."

To an outsider, doctors on rounds resemble priests as they gather around each infant in turn, muttering litanies of words and numbers, referring frequently to flow charts (in a nearby hospital, interns call them life charts) attached to the clipboards they carry like breviaries. However, their language sounds more like that of engineers at a space-launch station.

"I cranked up to 44 ccs on her, continuous infusions, cranked down on IV. TCs reading in the 50s . . ."

"Reduce fluid losses, monitor heart rate and mean arterial pressure. Go easy on fluids. See if we can come down on mean airway pressure . . ."

"His I-times may need adjusting. Try going up on rates; decrease the I-time." (Increase the frequency of ventilator-supplied breaths; cut down on inhaling time.)

"Is she still on the launch pad?" (The baby was to be moved to a smaller hospital closer to home.)

"Let's try it and see if he'll fly."

The pediatricians' training at Stanford involves returning to the ICN six times, twice as intern and four as resident, each time in a different capacity. On their first rotation they may work up to eighty hours a week, spending every third night on call. They learn the routines, collect various test results and measurements, write reports, and generally do what is known as scut work. They are overwhelmed with detail, overcome with anxiety, physically and emotionally exhausted. By the second rotation, they are somewhat enculturated and socialized. Things that shocked them no longer seem so terrible or bizarre.

Shortly after Dr. Molly Summers ended her first month in the ICN, shaken by what the infants were experiencing and what her participation in that experience might be doing to her, Dr. Carey Daggett ended her second rotation as intern. She felt more confident and enjoyed a newly won sense of power. She was more at ease with her earlier ethical doubts and no longer distressed over inflicting pain on the children.

"I got to flex my muscles more and learned more," she said, reflecting on her second month. "The decisions you make in the ICN are dramatic. That is what makes them interesting and controversial. When I was here last time the ethical questions bothered me a lot—much more than this time. I can see now that putting a two-year-old with a small chance of getting a kidney transplant on dialysis is no different from, say, saving a 750 gram infant. You have some abnormalities and a lot of kids who will be normal—kids who wouldn't have been without the ICN."

Enough ethical questions remained for Dr. Daggett to be uncertain whether she wanted to specialize in neonatology, but these pertained to outcome. While to Dr. Molly Summers the infants' suffering was a major source of personal anguish, it did not openly trouble the more experienced intern at all: "Of all the issues I deal with, whether or not I'm hurting a child is probably the least worry because I don't do anything that I don't think is necessary for their survival."

A certain amount of shutting off is essential to enduring the immensely demanding process of medical training, which is known to take a toll on house officers in depression, divorce, and a high incidence of suicide. But if a doctor treats a patient with only the goal in mind, dismissing the patient's experience, is that doctor a healer or a technocrat?

The values Dr. Summers had expressed were those Gilligan and others had linked with women. Concern with the patients' experience and her own relationship with that experience were central to her. Would she lose these concerns as she moved up the hierarchy? Was it desirable that she forswear empathy and shift her attention to life saving instead?

The definition of the word *compassion* is "to share suffering." Its antonym is *cruelty* or *inhumanity*. In the aboriginal traditions of Africa, Australia, and the Americas, the key to medicine lies in compassion. The medicine man or healer is required to take upon himself the sickness of the person seeking his help and then, ejecting it, set the patient on the way toward recovery. But the contemporary physician learns, during his or her training, to shut off emotion. Contemporary medicine demands distancing.

"One night, all night, I sat up with a four-year-old boy who was in septic shock," said the resident who found it hard to consider tiny preemies more than organisms and who plans to go into pediatric practice rather than neonatology. "I sat at the bedside all night. At six A.M., there was nothing more I could do. I watched the family go in to say good-bye. I started to bawl. The normal defense is to shut off the emotional aspect.

"The other day, I went to see *Terms of Endearment* [a film in which a young mother dies of breast cancer], and I could almost feel the glass wall going up. It was the protective barrier. As house officer you find that you need them. Without them you would become a total wreck and you could not deal rationally."

This resident is a gentle, sensitive man who was not completely at ease with the emotional distancing, even while recognizing that it was necessary. Both the physicians' training and the environment of the ICN demand it.[4]

The contemporary American physician embarks on his work without having had much opportunity for preparation other than academic and laboratory studies, followed by apprenticeship in the wards. Neither medical school nor internship and residency training teach the inner disciplines that help to cultivate self-knowledge and the ability to deal with the emotional stress of compassion. Distancing becomes a survival measure. It is ingrained in medical training and a natural consequence of the ICN environment. The real glass walls between the baby in the isolette and the doctor reinforce the glass walls in the mind. Consequently, even when physicians are the most humane and dedicated beings, the result can be the opposite of compassion.

As the young physicians move up the hierarchy into the profession, their job description changes and their enculturation continues. A senior resident reflected: "In the first year you are immersed in the details. In the second, you know what is going on and feel part of the decision-making process. This last, third, year you are with the attendings, helping them decide things. You do routine care, you have time to think. It is immensely more rewarding than the two prior years."

The main satisfaction he found during that last year was in terms of relationships with others on his team. "I felt I was able to make a comfortable, nonstressful experience for the interns. I made a specific point of helping them with scut work. It made their life enjoyable so that they were more of the team in a very dehumanizing experience." He also found he could monitor the rise of his own level of competence: "I tried to make decisions and then see how the attendings would decide—and found I was rarely wrong. So I learned something."

Residents seem to have a greater interest than interns in relationships on the team and a more acute awareness of their place in the hierarchy. "I'm at the highest level of the lower management or the lowest level of higher management," said one senior resident, describing herself.

After completing their residency, the pediatricians go out to practice—perhaps never to deal with fetus/babies again—or they pursue further specialization, in neonatology or another field. Dr. Richard E. Marshall, professor of pediatrics at the Washington University School of Medicine, has observed that people who choose to go into neonatology do so because they like the fast pace, intense treatments, and quick results. "In this regard, neonatologists often have aggressive and compulsive personality characteristics similar to that of surgeons, who also derive immediate rewards from the care of their patients."[5]

Some young physicians who aspire to a life as scientist/physician apply for fellowships, which at Stanford last three years. If accepted, they can combine clinical practice with research in a ratio of one to four. Much of the work at this particular institution relates to developmental biology.

By the time they are fellows, the young physicians have their own style of working; they are at ease in their competence. Although ethical issues still trouble them, they have arrived at a personal stance on many issues, including that of the ethics involved in using or refraining from aggressive treatment with very sick newborns. That stance will probably continue to change with time, and it will vary according to who they are and what they have experienced. This is true for all of their colleagues, even at the highest levels.

"If you wanted to interview ten of us today—and we could be from the same institution—you could have ten different attitudes, ranging over the spectrum," said Dr. Ariagno. "Some you would be very uncomfortable with because not enough would be done. Some would chill you because everything would be done when it is obvious that the chance of real benefit is close to zero."

When Dr. Ariagno decided to go into medicine, he had no idea that he might one day inhabit such a small, separate, and technology-laden world as the ICN. He grew up in a blue-collar town, Joliet, Illinois, where one of his models was the family doctor who gave free medical care, helped a community of nuns found a hospital, and came to the house to help his bewildered parents after his brother almost died from burns that covered 80 percent of his body.

"So my impression of practicing medicine had the aspect of a much wider job description than I currently carry," he said. "I was attracted to pediatricians in general because they could go into a room with an individual who couldn't give them a lot of information and find out what was wrong and be effective in helping.

"Then, when I came to the point where there was a lot of science involved with what I was doing, that was exciting, too. I still try to be a healer, scientist, teacher. I try to teach that it is possible."

Like other societies, the ICN has its peculiar rhythms and rites. The staff moves as an intricate clockwork, with interlocking teams of specialists changing according to their separate schedules, as a palace guard. The four neonatologists take month-long turns as attending and spend the months between their rotations on research, writing, lecturing, outreach to community practitioners, and travel to conferences all across the United States and abroad. The four neonatology fellows also change each month. They spend three-fourths of their time in research, one-fourth in the ICN, and have the greatest responsibility after the attending. Interns and residents rotate every month or six weeks, move on to the well-baby nursery, the pediatrics ward, nearby Children's Hospital at Stanford, and Santa Clara Valley Memorial Hospital in San Jose.

Meanwhile, the nurses and social support people remain at their stations, sometimes watching the doctors with tolerant amusement, sometimes clashing with them, usually working much more harmoniously than is the case in many other institutions. Everyone is on a first-name basis, and mutual respect prevails.

If the doctors, under the weight of their responsibility for numerous babies and the need to move rapidly from one emergency to another, do not have the opportunity to know most infants except as medical problems, the nurses become intimately acquainted with them and often form close affectionate ties. They see them more often than their parents do. They have no problem detecting when babies are in pain, when they dislike something, when they are pleased.

Nurses feel it is part of their role to remind the doctors that they are dealing with human beings rather than problems or assemblies of systems. "Sometimes they paralyze a baby so as not to blow out the lungs—and then they forget that the child is there," said one ICN staffer. Nurses try to protect the babies from avoidable intrusions. They speak up for babies when they think that a closer look at the course of treatment is indicated, and they frequently initiate group meetings with the physicians to discuss particular babies, especially those who are chronically ill and show no improvement.

More likely than physicians to view infants as unique individuals, nurses are also more likely to favor letting them go to spare them further pain. But if the infants start doing better, they are also immediately ready to coax them to carry on.

Many of the nurses empathize with the interns. Watching them progress is "like watching people grow up," said one longtime ICN nurse. "For many this is the most difficult and least liked rotation. It can be very ego-deflating." But they take issue when they think there is overtreatment. It seems to some of the nurses that physicians are so geared to action that they cannot bear to wait. They are not used to standing around. So they reach for morphine when a baby could be soothed by turning her to a position where she is comfortable, wrapping her so she feels safe, touching her quietly and with recognition.

"Often the problem is just environmental stress," said Darlene Allen, a respiratory therapist (RT) in the nursery who has special awareness of newborns because she had a sick baby who died. "You have to look at things in a mothering sense. I try to give them something that will remind them of the womb, that makes them feel held. There was this 800 gram baby—the TC was way up, the heart rate was down. I bundled him tight and he stabilized for the rest of the shift. You can put warm-water-filled balloons against them, or IV bags. Depending on what your job is, you may or may not notice these things. The nurses strive for them. I try. But it's extra time. Every RT's productivity is monitored. We have to chart minute by minute."

Thus, the technological aspect of the ICN society, which separates and dehumanizes, tugs against the caring aspect, which tries to nurture and heal.

While doctors, nurses, and respiratory therapists are engaged inside the ICN, just outside the nursery door, in a room with barely space enough for a long desk and two chairs, the three-person social support team works to help parents with their ordeal and future problems. The minuscule office is softly lit and almost always occupied. Every time a chair becomes empty, someone is likely to come in and sit down, for this cubbyhole is a refuge from the glare of the nursery. It is also an interface between the small separate society and the world from which the infants' families come and to which they return.

The social support staff say they have a bias: they believe that the baby belongs to the family. They find that doctors and nurses are apt to lose sight of that. Inside the ICN, parents are recognized as key participants, but they are, in a sense, aliens. Well-educated and affluent parents are likely to fit in and become part of the ICN society. In fact, some demand and obtain a more important role, relative to the treatment of their particular child, than the ICN staff would willingly yield. They know how to acquire power and wield it. But poor, uneducated, and culturally different parents tend to remain foreigners and to be suspect and misinterpreted, as happens to aliens everywhere.

It is significant, and indicative of the value the hospital places on correcting this injustice, that often a doctor cannot find a translator when he or she is conferring with parents on the gravest of issues. Housekeepers or relatives have been pressed into service. Since it is difficult, even in English, to explain what is happening in the strange environment of the ICN, inadequate translation can have dire consequences.

Social worker Charlene Canger remembers one Laotian family with whom the staff could not communicate. Only after she called people who were aware of Laotian culture did she realize why. For one thing, the staff had been praising the baby to help promote bonding between the mother and her child. They did not realize that, by so doing, they were calling the spirits' attention to the baby, risking having them take the baby back.

In addition, staff had spoken to the mother while looking directly at her, not knowing that eye contact was improper. The mother had kept looking away. And they had plunged into the subject without the polite neutral exchanges that are customary in many Asian cultures and that allow strangers to feel each other out. But worst of all, they had asked the mother about her sex life through a male interpreter and in front of the rest of the family, which included her husband and a very old lady. Only a woman, speaking privately, should have done that.

Grievous misunderstandings can result from linguistic or cultural misunderstandings, and all too often they pass unnoticed. Charlene Canger, who worked as a Peace Corps volunteer in the Philippines, is one of the few nursery staff members to have cross-cultural experience. With the Laotian family, she went out of her way to discover the problem. But pressures of time and other demands on attention do not always allow such inquiry.

Among the many specialists at the Stanford ICN, nobody is charged with serving as an intercultural interpreter. By contrast, expert and adequate help is provided in the billing office. A bilingual patient representative efficiently ensures that financial arrangements are in order, so that Stanford does not get stuck with the tab. Almost all bills are paid by third-party carriers, insurance companies, and state and federal aid programs. On any given day, someone in the hospital reception area can go to the computer and pull out an up-to-date account, to the penny, of what a baby's care has cost. ("Let's see . . I must have three to four million dollars up there now," a staff person with an account book said, running a finger down the ICN registrar. "The Monti twins, $79,000 A, $77,000 B; Maria Rodriguez, $112,665.85 . . ." She continued down the list of long-term tenants.)

But parent-staff misunderstandings can go unnoticed.

It is the job of the social workers to enfranchise parents as much as possible in the ICN society and to help them cope afterward. Researchers have shown that parents go through several distinct emotional stages after the birth of their premature or defective child. The first is grief, anger, shock, disbelief, and guilt. Then comes a search for reasons to be optimistic that the child will recover. Eventually, most parents come to terms with the situation and commit themselves to caring for their infant. The process may happen quickly, or it can be prolonged. Some parents hope against all hope for years.

The social support staff tries to help parents cope with the process, to find such assistance as they may need, and to introduce them to various groups and other parents like themselves. Aside from all that, the social support staff deals with an endless array of unique emergencies. Charlene Canger was doing all this, working part time and alone, until January 1982, when Kathy Petersen, having seen a need and deciding to fill it, appeared at the center with a plan.

Petersen is a physical therapist who then had twelve years' experience working with disabled children in the community. Over and over again, she had heard from parents that the one thing they wished they could have had, when they took their baby home from the hospital, was a little help in the transition, and in orienting themselves toward services that their neurologically and otherwise impaired children needed.

Bringing home even a normal baby from a nursery often is followed by a letdown. But bringing one home from the ICN, where the baby was special, subject of many kinds of attention, and the parents were special because they had a baby there, is inordinately more difficult. The special baby, once home, is just another baby—although harder to care for than most—and the parents are just parents. Most must cope alone with whatever arises. Public health nurses do visit, and some parents do call nurses they have come to know in the ICN, but the transition is tough.

Petersen approached Dr. Ariagno with her proposal. He was receptive, but told her that no funds were available for the work she envisioned. He suggested she try to raise some herself. So she wrote a grant proposal, obtained the medical center's approval, and approached a wealthy family whose child she had worked with at a center for the developmentally disabled after he had graduated from the Stanford ICN with cerebral palsy. The family agreed to back her and found three other contributors. A foundation was formed to fund Peterson for a year in her self-made job as discharge coordinator. Canger offered to share her undersized office, and before long Petersen was indispensable in the ICN.

Slim as a willow and athletic—she plays soccer on at least one team and sometimes on two—Kathy Petersen is friendly, vivacious, efficient, direct, and outspoken. Her views about intensive care for newborns have changed since her arrival at Stanford. She used to be very critical, working with damaged survivors. But at the center she has seen babies she never believed could survive go home to their families and return for ICN reunions looking perfectly normal. This experience has given her a new respect for the resilience of human beings.

The two subcultures in the intensive care nursery—the doctors and the nurses and social support staff—often oppose each another. Sometimes the goal of saving lives and the sense of compassion demand different paths of action and create a struggle of ends versus means. The borderline infants' survival requires that they endure an unknown quotient of pain. Assuming that an infant has a good chance of emerging alive, how much pain can be justified on the ground of the outcome? Is there a limit to what one may do to a child for the sake of saving its life?

The same questions have arisen with respect to adults under extreme stress: people who sought to commit suicide because they felt unable to bear any more pain; burn victims whose treatment was so excruciating they pleaded to be allowed to die rather than undergo it. In April 1974, Dax Collins, a twenty-six-year-old man, was severely burned over his entire body in an accident in Texas. To prevent infection, he was immersed daily in a Hubbard tank of saline solution. He repeatedly pleaded that the treatments cease, that he be permitted to die, even though his chances of survival were good. A year later, having been discharged from the hospital blind, with stumps instead of hands, and maimed from the contractures (resistance to muscle stretch) in both legs, he said he was glad to be alive. But he also said that he believed that someone who was suffering what he had suffered should be permitted to choose to die.

The question of whether the ends justify the means has occupied philosophers for many centuries. It does not seem to arise for most of the physicians we interviewed. They are dedicated to saving lives, and these violent, painful means are all they have at their disposal. In a way, neonatology is at a stage similar to that of dentistry when teeth were pulled out with pliers. The neonatologists' ethical battleground is not means, it is outcome.

"If the children all came back to the follow-up clinic with behavior problems, then I'd feel differently," said one of the attending physicians. "If we had a bunch of autistic or destructive children, then I would really be concerned. If behavior problems were the prominent thing reported in centers around the United States, then I think we'd have to take a look at it [the issue of

73

pain.] If every individual came through lacking the psychosocial development that would allow them to be effective human beings, that would be horrendous. But that does not seem to be the case. Our suspicion is that the infant person at least can pack the experience away somewhere in the psyche and that it is not very conscious."

The follow-up data is too scanty to show what, if any, the long-range harm might be. But even if the convenient assumption that the infants will forget totally is correct, does that justify everything? Does that make it all right to expose a totally defenseless human being—who usually cannot even protest by crying—to what might well be called torture if it were not therapy?

The question of means troubles many of the nursing and social support staff. "You see them, once recovered, happy. Their parents are happy. But every step has to mean something," said a nurse. "The more complex our technology becomes, the wider the gap between what is happening and our own ethical feelings about it." For her, the work in the ICN sometimes violates the Christian principle that life is sacred, not because babies die but because the means used to save them are so violent.

The infants in the newborn nursery cannot be heard on the matter, and nobody else really knows what they experience. How pain is factored into the choices made about treatment depends, to some extent, on the values of the individual physicians. Neonatologists seem to accord greater value to the alleviation of pain than do surgeons. The fact that they do leads them to search for ways to give morphine and seek to manage whatever side effects it may involve.

It may turn out that means and ends cannot really be separated, the one shaping the other, and that we will eventually realize that there is a price to be paid for life saving through such means as now exist.

Despite many differences in attitudes and values, the entire staff in the ICN is committed to the belief—backed by research evidence—that the benefits of the work under way here, for the infant population as a whole, far outweigh any costs. The entire staff is also frequently troubled by those instances in which the issue is in doubt.

Part Two

Acting and Reacting on the Medical Frontier

CHAPTER FOUR

A Miracle Baby:
The Way It's Supposed
to Work

The first time Peter Shaw entered the long, bright room he was on the run, hurrying alongside the team that had delivered the first of his twin daughters. He was wearing a pastel gown and mask, and his eyes were glued to the baby as, covered with a small plastic blanket, she was wheeled down the hall in a bassinet equipped with an overhead radiant warmer. She was twelve inches long and weighed 540 grams (1 lb. 3 oz.) and she was three months premature for a pregnancy that had begun in October 1983. One of the physicians had told him that only 10 percent of babies her size make it out of the delivery room and that for those who do, the chances are about fifty-fifty. Peter was crying as he ran.

When the team pulled into an unoccupied spot against the wall facing the window and clustered around the bassinet, Peter observed the lanky young physician in charge of this phase of the operation. His calm was reassuring. Surely it indicated that he had command of the situation. Peter watched the doctor lean over the small purple-red shape on the hotbed to attach a line to the umbilical cord. This was Dr. Michael Trautman, he would later learn, one of the postdoctoral fellows in neonatology who were next in command to the attending physicians.

Dr. Trautman looked up at the distraught father and, without stopping his work, began to explain, in an ordinary, calm voice, what he was doing.

"This IV is going into the belly button because it is an easy place to put an IV. There are no nerve endings in the umbilical cord so this does not hurt her. It goes way in to feed her, give her sugar, salt, take some samples of the blood so we can see how much oxygen she is getting. We can turn it up or down. We won't feed her now in the usual way. For now she will need this. These monitors are attached to see how she is doing," he said, pointing at lines that ran from pads that had been placed in several places on her body. "The temperature probe is to see if she is too hot or too cold. She will need this ventilator for a while." He gestured with his chin at the twin tubes that ran from a complicated machine to a narrow tube that had been inserted into the baby's throat. "See, the arms and fingers and toes are all there. Given the opportunity she will pull everything out so we will probably have to restrain her a little with gauze. She'll be in the hospital as long as she would have been inside her mom, probably. It's too early to talk about a lot of her problems. We hope she doesn't develop complications."

Peter was not taking in many of the particulars. But he saw, clearly, that this doctor, despite his apparent youth, was behaving like a competent laboratory scientist. This soothed him. Had something been seriously wrong, surely Dr. Trautman would be upset. Peter turned back to the delivery room.

It was only later, when the second girl, an ounce heavier than the first, had been installed in the nursery and Jacqueline was waking from her drugged state that Peter came back to take a real look at the place that he would later describe as his "life magnet."

When the Shaws had decided to have another baby, they had assumed it would be through natural childbirth, in this same hospital. There was no reason, at first, to think that would not be possible. Jackie was thirty-four and in good health. Their first daughter, Siena, had weighed five and a half pounds at birth and came only five days early. Although there had been a complication in that pregnancy—the placenta had separated and six weeks before the due date the baby had stopped growing—their obstetrician had assured them that this was not a problem they had to expect would recur with later babies.

They had wanted at least one more child. Peter came from a family of five siblings. Jackie, who was one of nine, thought maybe, if she managed all right with the next one, she might want yet one more. They had talked things over and made plans. The small two-bedroom house near downtown Palo Alto could be expanded by adding one more room. Peter's landscape architecture firm was doing well, and they could manage the financing. They applied for a bank loan, which was approved.

Five months into the pregnancy, Jackie fell ill, and everything was put on hold. The first indication was a finding of protein in her urine, observed during a routine visit to the Midpeninsula Health Service, an unusual prevention- and home care—oriented health plan to which they belonged. It stresses patient education, provides special phone-in times to doctors, and offers home visits. The finding of spilled protein led to a diagnosis of pre-eclampsia (toxemia), a complication of pregnancy that afflicts 5 to 7 percent of pregnant women. It brings high blood pressure, rapid weight gain, and swelling from fluid retention. Left untreated, it can develop into eclampsia, with seizures, brain hemorrhages, and coma.

A sonar scan showed that Jackie was carrying twins. This meant that the pregnancy was especially risky, for virtually every category of complication is increased significantly with twins. Risks include miscarriage, malformations, retardation, maternal and fetal hemorrhage, and premature delivery.

Later, the Shaws would attribute the twins' survival in large part to the quick and thoughtful action taken by their family physician, Dr. Patricia McGann at the service. She diagnosed the pre-eclampsia early and told them that it can sometimes be managed with bed rest and diet. She referred them to Dr. Gerald Shefren, an obstetrician who specialized in pre-eclampsia. As the condition was still at a very early stage, it had posed no serious hazard. It was possible, if they followed orders, maintained a positive outlook, and were lucky, that Jackie could continue to carry the babies until the seventh month, at least, when they would have an excellent chance of healthy survival.

Peter's mother, Mary Shaw, a nurse, was willing to help and to assume responsibility for the daily monitoring that would be required. Jackie was installed in her mother-in-law's law's house while Peter stayed home with Siena and took charge of getting her to nursery school and to friends' houses and of staying with her after he came home from work. His business was more than usually active at this time, but family always came first with him. Dr. McGann came daily at 7:30 A.M. to check on Jackie.

But Jackie's illness worsened, even with the special care she was receiving. So Dr. Shefren arranged for her admission to Stanford, where she could be treated for her rising blood pressure. She returned to Mary Shaw's home after two days, but not for long. During the ensuing month, she shuttled back and forth between home and hospital four times, becoming more weary and not improving. There was some danger now that the infants' growth would be retarded, because pre-eclampsia impedes the flow of blood to the fetus. Still, the Shaws and their physicians kept on with the effort to extend the pregnancy.

On April 10, 1984, at 11:00 A.M., Peter was at a client's home, discussing plans for a landscaping improvement, when his secretary called to tell him that his wife was at the hospital, in labor. He reached her side at 11:15, arriving moments before the obstetrician. Efforts to stop the labor with medication had been unsuccessful. The first girl was born at 1:08 P.M., the second at 1:14 P.M.

When he saw his first twin daughter—briefly, as she was being lifted up and handed to the team standing by—Peter was suddenly frightened. She looked like a little rat. She was so frail, not at all the baby that Siena had been. She was so very, very small. He realized that although he had prepared, he was not ready for this.

But as she emerged, he had heard one of the people standing by (two resuscitation teams, one for each baby, were ready) utter a sound of approval. "Nice delivery," someone had said. It had been a breech birth (bottom first), which is more difficult to deliver than the normal headfirst position. So perhaps it was all right. Peter's mind fastened to that, then returned to Jackie, who was struggling with the second baby. Her own mother had died in childbirth when Jackie was only ten. Did these doctors know? Should he tell them to be careful? He spotted the anesthesiologist conferring with another physician, a cardiologist perhaps, and hurried up to offer them whatever information might be relevant. But the physicians turned to him with what he perceived as cold unwelcome. Bristling a bit, he withdrew. At that point, the obstetrician said, "Dad, you'll have to leave." Anesthesia was now required. Peter saw the team leaving with the bassinet and fell in alongside.

Meanwhile, Mary Shaw was standing in the hall, very troubled. Unlike Peter, she was not thinking just of the babies' survival, she was worrying about something that could be worse than death. Such tiny babies did not necessarily die. Some of them grew up with mental impairment, cerebral palsy, damaged lungs, and other disabilities that doomed them and their families to a lifetime of suffering. She worried about her son and daughter-in-law, and about their sweet, spunky little Siena as well.

As the team came through the swinging doors from the delivery room and moved past her, she did not even recognize Peter, with his beard and lower face hidden behind a surgical mask, until he called out to her, "They don't even know yet if they will live."

The twins were on the threshold of viability in terms of weight, but they had an advantage over some others their size because they were small for their gestational age. The youngest babies to survive are born at twenty-four weeks, sixteen weeks short of the time the human being normally requires in the womb. Below twenty-four weeks, all the intensive care technology is generally useless, for the lungs are simply too immature to work. Jackie Walker-Shaw had managed to carry her twins into the twenty-seventh week, providing them with a vital margin of hope. But it was still a very narrow margin.

When both girls had been installed in the nursery, it occurred to Peter that it was vital to name them, immediately. They must not go another minute as Walker-Shaw A and Walker-Shaw B. They needed identities so they could be people. He and Jackie had agreed that their middle names should be after the two grandmothers, Mary and Miriam. And they had selected Angela as one girl's name. So the first would be Angela Mary. The second could be Yvonna—Jackie's mother had been named Yvonne—Yvonna Miriam. He would have to get his wife's approval.

He found that Jackie was still drugged. He could not get her to focus sharply enough to convey to her the importance of choosing a name that very moment. She emerged from her fog, however, just long enough to nod agreement. Peter hurried back to the nursery to inform the nurses.

Then he stood beside Angela, who was under a little transparent plastic tent, with an array of plastic tubes attached to the umbilical catheter, an endotracheal (ET) tube in her mouth, attached to two corrugated plastic hoses—one blue, the other white—that connected with the ventilator looming beside her. This raw fetal form, trapped by the life-sustaining web, was, at this moment, the center of his whole world. A nurse stepped back a bit to allow for such meager privacy as was possible in this setting. "Hi, Angela," Peter said. "Recognize my voice, huh?" His voice was laden with inchoate emotions that included fear, excitement, and anger. But the strongest note in it, piercing shakily through all the rest, was resolve. "You're a brave girl, Angela. Daddy loves you, Angela. I'm going to see Mommy now."

For the uninitiated it would seem that surely this man was ignoring the obvious. How could this unready being, this newborn who resembled a fetus far more than a normally born baby, hear and respond to this large person's loud words? Surely it was fanciful, even illusory, to think that any communication could have taken place. But at that particular moment, Peter Shaw had sealed his commitment. This was one of his two daughters. He had given them names. He was willing them to live, with all the determination he was able to summon.

And Angela did live, becoming one of those legendary babies who beat the odds. Hers is a story in which everything necessary was provided and everything worked. It shows what neonatology can do under the best of circumstances.

Angela Mary Walker-Shaw stayed in the intensive care nursery for the next seven and a half months. While her sister Yvonna grew stronger and larger, becoming what the physicians refer to as a "grower and feeder" who can do without their elaborate ministrations, Angela languished, contracting infections and other afflictions that kept her on the edge of survival week after week. Outside the drawn pink and yellow curtains, the spring rains ended, summer came and went, then maples turned red and dropped their leaves. The autumn rains began. Medical students finished their training and went on; others arrived. After three months and ten days, Yvonna Miriam went home where she did well.

Angela saw none of this. Her world, all this time, was the long, bright room with mechanical sounds, where neither night nor day nor seasons existed. She might as well have been inside a space capsule or somewhere deep underground. She saw no sun, no sky, none of the natural world except the adults who moved past her, stopped to inspect her and do things to her, and the parents who longed to touch her and hold her, but for a long time could not.

At first the twins' skin was so delicate that it was likely to tear when the surgical tape that kept needles and tubes in place was removed. Their limbs had no tone and flailed like the limbs of rag dolls. They had no protective muscle or fat and had not yet developed the heat regulation system that all warm-blooded mammals must have to survive. Deprived so suddenly of the warm, fluid-filled softness that had nourished them for six months, exposed now to the harsh light and air they could not yet tolerate, they would quickly have expired anywhere but in this kind of nursery.

They could survive in the intensive care nursery because radiant overhead warmers, then isolettes, (incubators) supply from without the heat they cannot yet generate within. To keep them from shriveling in this external heat, like fruit on the rack of a dryer, various fluids are infused through tubes attached to the umbilical line. Nurses, doctors, and technicians undertake to continue mechanically what had been happening mysteriously and naturally, beyond humankind's full understanding, within the mother. The prematurely ejected babies become subjects for medical engineering. Fluid and gas intakes and outputs, their composition, volume, and frequency, are meticulously measured. When something does not conform to the range of normalcy, steps are taken to compensate. Because blood samples are required frequently to determine how oxygen is diffusing, the extracted blood is replaced by repeated transfusions.

After two or three weeks, the umbilical line has to be abandoned. Leaving it in too long can cause infection. From then on, blood samples are taken by heel stick. This procedure bruises the minuscule heels and causes them to turn bluish-purple. Medicines and nourishment are injected through IVs, intravenous lines inserted in wrists, arms, and the scalp. After a while, as in hard-core heroin addicts, the babies' veins become so damaged by these repeated needle punctures that doctors must try for a long time before they find a spot that will accept the injection. Sometimes (as happened with Chris Lew and would eventually happen with Angela), in tiny babies who stay in intensive care for extended periods, no more usable veins can be found. The physicians have to call a surgeon to do a cut-down: a surgical incision, usually at the side of the neck, to a vein. The surgeon then inserts a central line, a catheter that runs down into the atrium of the heart. This central avenue works for monitoring, intravenous feeding, and medications, unless it becomes infected, which it is likely to do.

When Jacqueline recovered from the anesthesia she eased herself into a wheelchair and, escorted by a nurse, made her way down the hall and past the swinging doors marked Premature Infant Nursery. She stood up to look at her babies and felt faint. Fear cut her breath. She might have fallen had it not been for the wheelchair behind her. She would not return without Peter for some days.

Back in her room, she had time to think, but her imagination did not stretch to understand what she had seen. She felt empty. Her belly, which had not grown enough, was flat. Before she had fully appreciated her pregnancy, it was over. And out there were these two, red and scrawny, in a tangle of tubes and wires. They were not ready. How was she to mother them? She should have held them, held on to them somehow, kept them from being ejected. What would happen to them? To them, to her, to Peter and Siena? What was mothering in this situation?

Jackie had done plenty of mothering when her own mother had died, leaving her daughter, the third-eldest of nine, to tend to the younger brothers and sisters in Port of Spain, Trinidad. There, large families were the norm and were not confined to one home but stretched to include multiple cousins, aunts, and godparents all over the neighborhood. It was easier for a girl to grow up without a mother there than it would have been in a North American city, than it might have been for Siena. The possibility that she could have died of eclampsia was not one Jacqueline had allowed herself to entertain. Yet she could not entirely banish it from her mind.

As she lay in her hospital bed, confused and grieving, trying to grasp what had happened, her mind roamed her past. Somehow, the pieces would fit back together. The twins were alive. Babies that size survived and grew to be normal, healthy people. She had read it; she had been told. There were risks, but there was also hope. One had to think positively. Great medical breakthroughs had been made in recent years. Women did not hemorrhage to death in childbirth at a medical center like this one, and things that defied common sense and experience were possible.

In Trinidad, even today, these babies would have died. Everyone would accept it and everyone would come to mourn. They would bring food and they would sing. It had been that way after her mother's death. There were no secrets and you were not alone. Everyone knew you from the time you were born. Now, despite all her husband's concern for her, Jacqueline felt cut off from all she knew.

Her illness had weakened her spirit. Her normal self was a person who looked reality straight in the eye and stood up to it. Jackie had learned to make her own way in life, having been raised to be strong. But she would have to let some time pass before she could gather the courage to return to the babies.

At first, it seemed that Yvonna was the twin in more serious trouble, for she had severely collapsed lungs. Angela soon was breathing on her own, and when she was thirty-six hours old, the breathing tubes were removed from her. Whether this was a good idea was, at the time and in retrospect, controversial among the ICN physicians. Because of the hazard of chronic lung disease for small premature babies, some physicians try to take out the tubes as soon as possible, to prevent ventilator dependency. But others wait longer, reasoning that the effort to breathe takes too high an energy expenditure for the tiny infants. There is insufficient data to allow either view to prevail as more sensible.

While her sister's condition stabilized, Angela experienced a stormy first few days. Her heart stopped three times, and she recovered only after major resuscitative efforts. On the third day, a sonar scan of her head showed that she had a grade II intraventricular hemorrhage, the severity bordering on grade III. Such brain bleeds, graded I to IV in severity, are common with very premature babies, whose extremely fragile capillaries are easily injured. Brain damage may result. In Angela's case, an electroencephelogram taken when she was one week old showed no specific abnormalities, and that was a promising sign.

Then infection set in. Angela became very pale and her stomach swelled. Dr. Ariagno called Peter at home at about 2:00 A.M. to tell him that it was touch and go. Peter had come down with a horrible cold the day after the birth, the strain of the past weeks finally having found a release, and this news did not help his condition.

Angela had developed necrotizing enterocolitis (NEC), a gangrene-like infection of the gastrointestinal tract that afflicts some premature infants, particularly those of very low birth weight whose immature gut fails to withstand severe stress. The disease was first described in the 1960s, when very small preemies were beginning to be saved, and for the ensuing decade was a scourge in the intensive care nurseries. About three-fourths of the infants who contracted NEC died. Since then, both the incidence of NEC and its death toll had dropped sharply.[1] In this ICN, it was now rare.

In babies with NEC, bowel function is disturbed, the intestines fill with gas, and the belly becomes distended. The baby vomits, has diarrhea, may suffer from respiratory distress, below-normal body temperature, and sepsis, a blood infection. In advanced cases, the intestinal walls occasionally perforate, allowing the normally harmless bacteria that live in the intestine to invade the tissue and cause infection.

Treatment with antibiotics failed to clear up the condition for Angela. On the eighth day, it was clear she had succumbed to NEC to the point where her intestines had perforated. The Shaws were informed that surgery would be required. The damaged and dead portions of the intestine would be removed in a procedure called a resection. The severed ends would be brought to the surface temporarily. The upper part of the intestine would have to do all the work of fluid and food absorption until the two parts were reconnected.

At the same time, the surgeons would cut another opening, through the abdominal cavity into the stomach and fit in a tube. The baby would be fed through this gastrostomy if problems occurred in the normal route.

Angela weighed only 460 grams at this point. Like most infants, she had lost some weight after birth. There were risks to the procedure on an infant so small. Would she survive anesthesia? The added insults? Would enough intestine be left for her to be nourished? If not, she might become permanently dependent on intravenous feeding, which would work only for so long.

Although the risks were serious, the physicians did not believe the baby would survive without the surgery. So, on the eighth day of Angela's life, fourteen inches of dead tissue—up to a third of her total intestine—were removed.

One of the surgeons at the center who, like the other physicians, divides his time between clinical service and research, remarked, "She is probably the smallest and youngest baby to have this major an abdominal operation. Her father asked me if she was the smallest I had ever operated on and I said she was the smallest *human*, but that my rats are much smaller. My rats weigh an ounce." Remembering Peter's reaction, he added, "There are probably times when it is not right to be totally honest."

Angela was fed breast milk directly into the gastrostomy. But as she now had only two thirds of the intestine she had had before the surgery, the milk ran through it quickly and was only partially absorbed. She gained a little weight, then lost again. On July 10, when she was three months old, she weighed only 1110 grams (2 lbs. 7 oz.). Because she was so very small and frail, she picked up infections in the nursery: a respiratory syncytial virus, in which cells in the lung form clumps and for which there is no treatment; Klebsiella, a bacterial infection that affects respiration and the urinary system; a staphylococcus infection.

At the beginning of August she seemed to be doing well enough for her gut to be reconnected soon. The surgeons thought that could be done when she reached 1500 grams. After that, it was anticipated, she could go home. Since Angela now seemed to be a grower and feeder, she was transferred into the intermediate nursery. But the nurses there began to report that she was refusing to eat or throwing up her food. Back she went to the main nursery.

The treatment of such minuscule humans is still so recent that much of what happens to them is fortuitous, a best guess, intuition. Often, treatment for one condition causes troubles elsewhere. The physicians wield powerful tools on delicate organisms. It is as though they had only hacksaws, machetes, and high-pressure hoses to work with in a greenhouse full of orchids. They do the best they can, always acknowledging, however, that there is a great deal that they do not know.

"This is what's so hard," Peter Shaw later reflected. "Things happen, and often the doctors don't know why. They ask your consent, but you really have no choice. The children are yours, but you really have no power, because they are basically the staff's babies. We would have preferred not to have the surgery and I would have preferred not to have Angela extubated so soon. They don't know whether it traumatized her or contributed to her infection. The more you're around there the more you realize they don't know. And when you realize that, that opens up that much more questioning."

Peter questioned a lot. And doctors, with many other patients to consider, were not always glad to discuss the details of treatment. Once, Peter said, a senior physician, whom he had not yet met but who apparently had heard of Peter's inquisitiveness, introduced himself and said sarcastically, "Mr. Shaw? Or is it *Dr. Shaw?*"

The physicians were as exasperated with Peter as he was with them. They felt that he failed to understand some basic facts about intensive care units: that they were highly dangerous places for adult, child, or infant; that the physicians are never totally in control of the dilemmas that evolve; that no recipe exists for doing things correctly; and that the list of problems that must be solved moment to moment is endless. "Some families would like to take charge, take the medical role," said one of the doctors. "But that is as impossible as it would have been for them to take Angela home after birth and apply herbal medicine as the primary care."

The risks for threshold-viable babies like Angela are so great, this doctor said, that when one did well, he was awed. Peter, however, seemed not to understand the enormity of the odds that had to be overcome if his children were to survive undamaged. It seemed to this doctor that Peter's attitude was a form of arrogance, even a form of playing God.

A recent study of parents in an intensive care nursery found that fathers are sometimes more comfortable than mothers in the situation. The reason: they can understand that work is under way. They tend to appreciate the action, the challenge, and to be more at ease with the technology.[2]

To combat his feeling of helplessness in the nursery, Peter resorted to a kind of magic. He found himself compulsively conducting little private rituals. He became superstitious about coming every day at a particular time. When he washed his hands he always cleaned under his fingernails, ritualistically. He was superstitious about how he drove to the hospital, how he parked the car, how he walked in. Later, when he looked back on that time, he said, "I never told anyone all this. But it was the kind of thing that had worked for me in sports. I had always been involved in

sports—football and baseball and later handball. My competitive-
ness and this kind of attitude probably had a lot to do with my
commitment to the twins, too. I guess I was sort of a fanatic. And
the nurses thought I was nuts. But I was successful in sports. I
guess if you have a certain method and consistency, it pays off."

Nobody will ever know whether Peter's magic made any difference to Angela. Certainly her parents' devotion to her did. Everyone in the nursery knows that, beyond the technology and the
treatments, it is often the intangible human factors that turn the
hand of fate for the babies. Angela was fortunate, not only in her
parents, but also because she lucked into intelligence, care, and
love in the nursery. A number of people went out of their way to
look out for her.

Dr. Philip James, twenty-nine, was the fellow on duty the night
Angela became very sick, and he had an idea that may well have
made a life-and-death difference for her. He decided to give her a
transfusion of white cells to help her fight her infection. But because it was late and the lab that supplies the blood was not open,
he decided to transfuse from the mother, who was still in the hospital. It would not only help the baby, he thought, it might be a
nice thing for the parents, a chance for them to make a positive
contribution to their baby instead of just watching helplessly.
Jacqueline's blood helped Angela make it through a critical night.

Michael Trautman was on the day of the operation. He had developed a special interest in Angela, as tends to happen when a
physician is called on to pay special attention to some baby. He
had not only been there for the delivery, he had also worried over
her when she was extubated. Now he was concerned that the
anesthesiologists might not have adequate experience with babies that small, so he did something that the fellows in the ICN
do not usually do; he went to surgery with her and stood by.

Decisions about Angela were made daily by a sizable number of
people. Many of them came and went, on rotating schedules. But
throughout it all there was continuity, thanks largely to her primary nurses, especially Gayle Hand.

Not all babies are lucky enough to have consistent primary
nurses. Though an effort at continuity is made, reassignment is
often unavoidable as the needs of particular babies and of the
nursery change. Not infrequently, however, a nurse becomes especially committed to a particular baby. When that happens, she
does everything in her power to stay with that infant. She gets to
know the baby intimately and gives him the most special care,

beyond the excellent care that she normally gives. She would not say so because that would be unprofessional, but she comes to love the baby.

Gayle Hand is warm and ample. An infant fits into her arms with utter ease. The roundness of her face is emphasized by her round glasses; her long hair is pulled together casually at the nape of her neck and hangs down her back. She emanates motherly femininity. This was her ninth year in the ICN. She had become interested in newborn intensive care while she was still a nursing student, when a cousin suffering from lupus gave birth to a baby that was small for gestational age. Like most of the nurses in the Stanford ICN, she was satisfied with her choice of specialty. "It's rewarding," she said, "the intensity, the excitement, the chance to work one on one with babies. There are so many advances being made."

Usually, Gayle tried to keep her work and her private life separate. When she left the hospital, she tried to leave her involvements. She lived alone with two cats, Midnight and Kitty, and she had her workday routine down to clockwork.

On the day the twins were born, Gayle was the transport liaison nurse, making arrangements and keeping records on new babies coming in from the delivery room and from other hospitals. She had finished her paperwork and was just about ready to go home when the twins were born so precipitately. On impulse, she volunteered to take one of them.

"Angela was the A twin. Usually the B twin is sicker, so I said, 'I'll take A,' she recalled one day in September, when Angela was five months old. "She seemed mature for her size. Her skin didn't fall off when you touched her. That I find hard, when even touching them damages them.

"When she was about a week old she had an episode that required resuscitation. The endotracheal tube became dislodged. It happens. They get this gray-green pasty look. Then her abdomen became bloated, gray and discolored. I thought she was going to die. At the time, it wasn't upsetting to me. Some babies make it, some don't. But now I feel differently. I've never felt the attachment I've felt for this baby. I've felt the responsibility. But this is beyond what I am knowledgeable in."

She knew the exact moment when her feelings had changed. It had happened two months earlier, on a slow day. A baby was about to be transported back to the hospital it had come from, a three-hour drive away. Angela had been fine all day, so Gayle volunteered.

When she returned the baby was flailing about. She had been screaming, other nurses told her, the entire time Gayle was gone. The moment Gayle was at her side again, saying, "Angela, what is the matter?" she opened her eyes and relaxed. Gayle was astonished: Angela knew her.

"I'd always said, 'I'm here a hundred percent when I'm here, but when I'm home, don't call me in the middle of the night.' I always felt that I should be able to go home and leave this. The nurses are loving as well as expert. But they don't expect anything back. But here was interaction. Angela gave something back."

All along, but especially since that crucial moment, Gayle felt that the baby initiated suggestions about ways she could be helped to eat and grow. At first, after the operation, her food was dripped into her gastrostomy. At about two or three months, when Angela was 1000 grams, Gayle felt that the infant wanted to suck, so she offered her some breast milk through a nipple and gave her a pacifier, which she seemed to like. It satisfied a need and calmed her. Gayle told other nurses about it and they followed her example. Angela continued to make progress.

But one day, she suddenly refused to eat, turning her head away and crying when milk touched her mouth. A septic workup was performed, because feeding intolerance is the first sign of infection. Gayle felt the pangs of guilt nurses typically feel when infection occurs. Though they know it cannot be totally prevented, they always worry whether, somehow, they might have neglected a precaution.

What troubled Angela was not an infection. Gayle realized that after she had taken a five-day vacation. When she had returned she found that not only was Angela not eating, she had changed in an odd way. She stared, bug-eyed. She was likely to startle, to vomit, and to arch her back and breathe erratically. She would turn away from the bottle and also from people's eyes.

So Gayle began to think that perhaps this was a behavioral problem. She recalled that during her residency at Mount Zion Hospital in San Francisco, while she was working toward a master's degree, she had seen a chronically sick baby who would not eat. In that case the problem was found to have been lack of affectionate contact. The nurse would feed that baby in the isolette without holding her. In Angela's case, there was no shortage of loving concern. Gayle and the other primary nurse were devoted to Angela, the parents came daily, and the grandmother also visited often, independently. Still, Gayle knew she was on to something.

She also recalled that Dr. Peter Gorksi at Mount Zion, a pediatrician who specialized in the development of high-risk infants, had observed that premature babies, at a certain phase of their development, do not habituate to stimuli. They respond and keep responding until the result is stimulus overload and a physiological state of hyperalertness, a state in which the infant is especially vulnerable and which is not compatible with easy food intake.

Gayle observed that Angela was subject to constant intrusions. Her crib was in a heavily trafficked section of the nursery. She had been there so long that a lot of people knew her. She no longer looked like a fetus, as so many of the other infants did. She was a baby. It was possible to interact with her. So almost everyone did, continuously. Could she be suffering from overstimulation?

In addition, a string of different nurses had cared for her on one of the shifts. Her father's dedication to her took a form that some of the staff found difficult to work with. He would say things like "That's a clean gown, isn't it?" or "Don't you think it's a good idea to wash your hands before you touch my daughter, if you have been using the phone?" Some of the nurses took remarks like that so badly that they avoided assignment to Angela. One nurse had even had a nightmare in which Peter had been yelling at her because he had come in and found that Angela had been moved.

Gayle mentioned her stimulus overload theory to Dr. Ariagno, who thought it worth investigating and suggested that Dr. Gorski be invited for a consultation—an unusual step. Meanwhile, to assure that the infant had some nourishment, a central venous line was put in: a catheter, inserted into a vein through a surgical cut at the neck, running into the right atrium of the heart, where circulation is rapid and the chance of infection is lessened. A solution containing essential proteins and other nutrients (TPN— total parenteral nutrition) dripped through the line. Additional nourishment was dripped into the gastrostomy. Angela could not refuse to be fed now. But she continued to refuse to nipple.

Awaiting Dr. Gorski's visit, Gayle took some steps on her own to provide the peace and quiet that she felt the baby needed. She put up a hand-lettered sign: "Please let Angela get her sleep. Do not wake unless absolutely necessary." She backed up the parents, who had asked repeatedly that Angela be moved to a quieter location, out of the flow of traffic. And she continued a practice Mary Shaw had begun, draping the bed with a blanket when Angela slept.

The consultation with Dr. Gorski attracted much interest among the nurses, physical therapists, and social workers. No specialist in development was on the Stanford nursery staff. A crowd gathered to hear the consultant's observations. The only other physician present, however, was a house officer newly arrived on rotation. Some staffers took this as evidence of lack of interest among Stanford doctors in how the human and physical environment affects infants. However, there were many possible explanations for other physicians' absence.

Dr. Gorski recognized in Angela a pattern of neurodevelopmental disorganization common among premature infants hospitalized in intensive care units for a long time. He observed that Angela was maturing. Normally, a baby at three months of age begins to sleep longer periods at night and stay awake longer by day. She becomes less fussy, starts to vocalize with open vowel sounds, and plays with hand-eye coordination. A great deal of cortical reorganization is going on. It is a time of some stress.

In addition to this normal organic stress, Angela was experiencing the heavy stress of the environment. She was bombarded with stimuli in the busy, noisy nursery. She had almost no means to control these, except by turning away, avoiding eye contact, and rejecting food by refusing to nipple or throwing up.

Dr. Gorski suggested several ways to change Angela's self-destructive behavior. He recommended that her physical environment be modified to expose her to fewer stimuli; that the surgical reconnection of her intestines be postponed to give her a chance to settle down; that the nursing care be kept as consistent as possible; that the parents be brought into the process and helped to understand her condition.

The entire report, but most particularly a recommendation that Dr. Gorski made toward the end of his report on the visit, was a vindication for Gayle. He urged, "Support the valiant nursing and physical therapy team in their devoted feelings of attachment and resultant heightened state of sensitivity, emotionally, to this child."

So the nurse's devotion to Angela was acknowledged to be all right. Gayle had at times felt apologetic about the intensity of her feelings, sensing that they might be thought unprofessional. But Dr. Gorski was saying it was all right to feel that way. Her affection for Angela had long ago broken through the dividers she had tried to keep between her work and her private life. She thought of the child in her leisure hours and sometimes went well out of her way to do things that might please her. Once she went to several stores in search of a nipple that Angela might prefer. Several times she wandered into toy shops for stuffed animals or other items that might be nice to look at or touch. She was bonded.

The day after the consultation, Angela was moved to a spot by the window in Room One, which was declared the quiet room. She could now look out at the trees blowing in the wind outside. The move meant that some of the nurses had to be reassigned: either Gayle or another RN had to change babies. Gayle, newly empowered, fought to stay with Angela and succeeded.

"It is very unusual for a baby to be here this long or clearly care who is taking care of her," she explained. "People think I have developed an attachment. But Dr. Gorski said she should be cared for by people she knows."

Peter and Jackie read the consultant's report and were angry. Why had it taken this man's recommendation to get Angela moved to a quiet room when they had repeatedly asked for just that, in vain? And, more important, why had the parents not been invited to the consultation? Peter felt that he and Jackie knew more about their baby than anyone else did, and he disagreed with some of the statements in the report. Some of the observations of Angela, as reported, were at variance with his own. He had been visiting his daughter daily and she had not turned away from *him*. Once again, he felt excluded from participation in decision making about his child. Whose baby was Angela, anyway? He phoned Dr. Gorski to express his concerns and to say he felt the parents should have been invited to the conference. The consultant agreed and said he had wondered why the parents were absent.

In the months that he had been making daily trips to visit Angela, Peter had gone through many personal changes. He had experienced disappointment with friends. "Most people stayed away. At first I was angry and felt I didn't want to have anything to do with anyone who did not make some kind of overture to us, but then I realized that few people understand or even attempt to. That made me reanalyze a lot of things. I really changed. There are always things one wants to do in life and puts off. I always had an interest in art, and I minored in art in college. But my job always came first. But four or five months after the twins were born I got a studio and started painting. In the midst of all this! There was an overriding need to get on with what I wanted to do with my life.

Of Angela's parents, Peter was the more regular visitor during all those months. Sometimes he came as often as three times in a day. Living only blocks away and working in the area, on his own schedule, he could do so. Jacqueline, busy at home with Yvonna and Siena, usually came once a day. While Peter had made Angela's survival a matter of triumphant determination, she was keeping her feet on solid ground and remembering that anything might still happen. It was almost as though, to protect herself and the other two daughters, she had to keep from getting too involved with the frailest baby until it was clear she would not die.

Angela grew. Finally, just before Thanksgiving, when she was seven and a half months old, she went home, and—although she was only half the size of her sister, who also was very small—she weathered the winter months without having to return to the hospital.

In April 1985, when Yvonna was beginning to walk and Angela, only eight and a half pounds, had learned to sit up, the Shaws gave a birthday party at Mary Shaw's house, to which they invited the people in the nursery who had played such a crucial part in their daughters' lives. Several nurses, including Gayle, attended. She had not seen Angela, the baby she had so grown to love, since her departure from the nursery, and she was a little afraid of her own emotions. Would the baby recognize her?

Peter handed the child to her so the man with the video camera could film them together. Gayle saw Angela look for her parents. She quickly returned her to Peter. Their relationship had ended.

On June 19, 1985, the Shaws brought their twin daughters to the clinic at Children's Hospital, where their development would be followed every six months until they were three years old, as part of a study on very low-birth-weight infants. Jackie held Yvonna; Peter carried Angela. Both had turned into charming mini-children. Yvonna continued to be the bigger and stronger, twenty-seven inches tall and weighing 6.5 kilograms (14 lb. 5 oz.);

Angela was twenty-three and a half inches and 4.5 kilograms (9 lb. 9 oz.). Developmentally, Yvonna was also ahead. Angela had just started to crawl and to pull herself up to standing. Both were tested by physical therapist Kathy Petersen, using the Bayley Scales, a standard measure for assessing mental, motor, and behavioral development in infants and small children. Angela had arrived at a stage appropriate for a one-year-old, if adjustment was made for prematurity. Yvonna was at fourteen months without adjustment. As she watched Angela playing with a bell, finding cubes under an upturned cup, and performing other tasks that show competence, Kathy Petersen was delighted. With more than fourteen years of experience in watching small children she could assure herself that both twins were doing amazingly well.

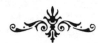

Angela became a miracle baby. She represents the amazing possibilities in a modern nursery. The fact that miracles like Angela do happen leads many people to expect that they can happen for anyone. It inspires everyone in an intensive care nursery to work very hard on babies born at the threshold of viability. When there is success, the effort seems heroic. When there is failure, the effort seems more than tragic; it seems to become almost torture. The odds for a happy outcome such as Angela's may be discouraging for most extremely low-birth-weight infants, but the existence of miracle babies serves as a beacon, leading doctors and parents to persevere.

It is important, therefore, to realize that in Angela's case there was a rare confluence of the best of possible circumstances. Her family was deeply committed to her and her sister and well educated and economically comfortable, able to devote much time to her in the hospital and at home, to secure the best in prenatal and post-hospital care, and had a very positive outlook. She was born in a hospital that was well equipped and well staffed for her care. She was delivered by a doctor who had been watching her mother's pregnancy and her own prenatal development. She was also lucky in meeting doctors and nurses within the hospital who went beyond the usual standards of care for her.

Many, if not most, premature infants are not born into such fortunate circumstances. Prematurity correlates with poverty, low education levels, teenage parenthood, problems such as alcoholism and drug abuse, and various family, social, and health problems. Babies who are born early into families with such problems are far less apt than Angela was to become miracle babies.

Babies like Angela are a joy to their parents and to all who helped them survive. But it is a mistake to use their existence to magnify the odds for all extremely premature infants.

The ICN is a confusing place, in every sense. Physically, it is incomprehensible to the layman. Philosophically, it is in turmoil. What decisions are made and by whom represents one of the greatest societal challenges we face. A success story like Angela's, where the near impossible becomes a reality, is success with two faces—promise and responsibility. Just as our society decided that it is better to free a hundred criminals rather than prosecute an innocent man, are we now deciding to force a hundred infants to live a tragedy so we might celebrate these wonderful babies? Are we actually deciding this, as a society, or is it being decided de facto, as the existence of life-support technology itself becomes a force dictating its use?

CHAPTER FIVE

When the Infant Decides

What leads some borderline infants to survive and others to die remains, even in the modern intensive care nursery, a mystery. Physicians and nurses often say that the babies decide. For they can sometimes see nothing specific that distinguishes a twenty-six-weeker who lives from one who succumbs. Some just seem to give up, they say, while others—Matthew Cordell, Jr., for example—are fighters.

Matthew Jr.'s conception defied the odds. Sophie had become pregnant despite the fact that she was equipped with an intra-uterine device (IUD), one of the most effective birth control methods. A sergeant in the navy, she was not at all eager to have another baby just then. But at the same time, she and Matthew, her husband, saw in the pregnancy an opportunity to save their marriage, which had been traveling a bumpy road for some time.

They had met in the navy. Sophie had joined with the express purpose of finding a husband, Matthew with exactly the opposite intention. "I came in vowing I would not get married until after I got out," he said. "I wanted to get some technical training and see the world, like they promise in the posters. That and an honorable discharge is all."

Sophie, who was high-strung and assertive, came from Texas, where she had been raised by her father and her strict, religious grandmother. Her teenage mother had left her and a sister, going on to have five more children elsewhere. Despite her grandmother's efforts to keep her away from boys, Sophie began to follow in her mother's footsteps, becoming pregnant and marrying at age sixteen. She finished high school at a special school for teen mothers and lived for four years with her first husband. Then the marriage fell apart and, at age twenty-two, Sophie enlisted. In the navy, Matthew's handsome looks, warm smile, and easygoing manner soon won her affections

Matthew intended to have a family, a large one, later. He had grown up as the youngest son in a family of nine, remembering that their needs had always been met, even though they lived in a part of town known as a ghetto, and that his holidays were always filled with plenty. His father, with all those children, had managed to earn a degree in accounting at night school and get a good job. When the baby of the family started school, Matthew's mother also had gone to work and they had moved to a suburb, so their children could attend better schools.

Eventually, Matthew thought, he would like to have seven children. "I don't know why, but that number, seven, was always in my mind." He married Sophie, and before their four-year enlistments were up they had a daughter.

Their relationship was programmed for trouble. Sophie was not at all thrilled by the idea of presiding over a vast family. What she relished was moving around in the world, learning new skills, holding down responsible duties outside the household. She also liked the navy and was proud of her advance in rank. So she wanted to stay in while he was eager to get out. They argued until she yielded.

Matthew was discharged first. He moved in with his parents near San Francisco while looking for a job and a house for his own family, now numbering four with his nine-year-old stepson and one-year-old daughter. With the skills he had acquired in data processing, he felt certain he would find well-paid work in the Silicon Valley.

But by the time Sophie came out, Matthew was still looking, so all of them stayed with his parents. Sophie found this arrangement unbearable, partly because her in-laws doted on their son but found many things to disapprove of in his wife. So one day, on impulse, she took an enormous gamble. She reenlisted. "I figured I would have an income and he could stay a civilian," she said.

But her plan misfired. Matthew found a job while she was sent several states away. After a short time, she applied for a discharge on the ground of hardship to the family. It was denied. Matthew appealed through every channel he knew, to no avail. So he decided their marriage was over. But then, the day after they said what they thought was a final good-bye, it occurred to Sophie that she might be pregnant. She had thought nothing about missing a couple of periods because, with an IUD, she was sure she was safe. Yet there were unmistakable symptoms. Indeed, she was three months along.

So Matthew Jr., while only a tiny fetus, became the reason for his mother's honorable discharge and the rescuer of his parents' disintegrating marriage.

A week before her discharge, Sophie started spotting. She went to the base hospital for a checkup, was given an ultrasound test, and was told that there did not seem to be anything to worry about. After she arrived in San Francisco, the bleeding increased. Another ultrasound, in a civilian hospital, showed a problem with the placenta: it was at the bottom of the uterus instead of on top. But during her next prenatal visit, to a military hospital, she was told it seemed normal. "I was using four to six pads a day, but the doctor said this was like having a period during my pregnancy," said Sophie. "Some women do."

Sophie found a job in San Francisco and, with Matthew, enrolled in some Saturday classes to improve her earning skills. She wanted to get as much as possible accomplished before the baby came. He was due in October. But he arrived in July.

The day before Sophie went into labor, she had another prenatal checkup and told the doctor she felt a cramp in her leg. He thought the baby might be pressing on a nerve. But that night the cramp tightened, the bleeding increased markedly, and she began to have contractions. Matthew drove her to the nearest military hospital, from which she was sent to the nearest community hospital, from which she was sent to Stanford, where, she was told, the delivery might be averted with medication.

But it was too late. Stanford doctors found that the placenta was, indeed, inserted low in the uterus and that this accounted for the bleeding. Nothing could be done to postpone the birth, nor was there any time to try to help the baby's lungs mature by administering steroids. Matthew arrived weighing 750 grams, just over one pound ten ounces. A doctor told his father that the baby was unlikely to live, but that they would just have to wait and see. Tiny Matthew was intubated and installed in the intensive care nursery.

At the time, nobody could predict what was to follow. Most preemies his size either expire soon or go home within three months or so. This one did neither. He became one of those children who most trouble doctors and nurses in the ICN because, under their ministrations, their lives keep flickering without either flaming or going out.

Matthew's story demonstrates some of the ethical dilemmas that confront those who work to save lives in the nursery. It is also a powerful example of the role the infants play in decision making.

Matthew contracted the familiar nursery ailments: respiratory distress, pneumonia, viral and bacterial infections. He recovered from each, but not quite enough to go on, grow, and get well. He was on the respirator, off the respirator, getting better, getting worse, "hanging in there," as one of the interns, with a resigned sigh, put it during rounds. His weight dropped to one pound five ounces, peaked to two pounds eleven ounces, then dropped to two pounds five ounces.

For a time he was known among the nurses as one of the Foursome: four chronically ill babies of about the same size, whose incubators were in a cluster at the end of the main room, all "hanging in there." One would die after months of lingering; one would go home with serious neurological problems but in better shape than the doctors had expected; and one would go home looking perfectly normal and healthy, even though she had been the smallest of them all, weighing 520 grams, slightly over one pound two ounces, at birth. Matthew outlasted them all as a nursery resident. Eventually he acquired a reputation as a kind of tiny hero, someone who refuses to give up.

The attending physicians rotated twice, packs of interns and residents came, went, came again, and saw with surprise that Matthew's name was still there, printed in red block letters on the roster at the nursery door. His person, not much larger than it had been in the previous months, still lay huddled inside. His rate of growth was slower than that of his chart, which bulged to a ponderous tome with X-ray results, lab reports, reams of prescriptions, and the scribblings of interns and nurses who saw him through repeated crises. Sometimes he was only a few breaths from expiring. But he pulled out from every setback, though just barely enough to go on.

At the very beginning, the ICN staff thought of Matthew as just another borderline-viable baby. Neither physicians nor nurses can afford to invest themselves emotionally with all patients. If they did, they would not survive their many losses. They are drawn in, however, as they get to know particular babies, as their personal experience with a tiny individual grows. They invest in the challenge of the baby's problem, with increasing intensity as their efforts begin to show success. And at times—as happened with Matthew—they also become involved with a baby as a person.

A senior resident said, "When I first saw Matthew, I thought, Oh, I've seen his kind before. But then, when he got better, I found myself rooting for him. I'm sure that when I'm back in two months, I'll still be asking what happened to Matthew Cordell."

His getting better was a matter of the occasional up among many downs. His main problem was a syndrome fairly common among babies of his degree of prematurity. It was iatrogenic, that is, caused by the treatment. The mechanical ventilation required to keep him alive had damaged Matthew's lungs. He seemed to be progressing inexorably toward bronchopulmonary dysplasia, a chronic lung disease in premature infants who have experienced severe respiratory distress and subsequently are treated with oxygen and ventilation. The lungs are so damaged that they no longer perform the essential function of ridding the blood of carbon dioxide and replenishing it with oxygen. On an X-ray, they look like Swiss cheese. The architecture of the alveoli (air sacs) is disrupted, the tissue is collapsed, dense in some places and irregularly perforated in others. The longer the baby stays on the respirator, the harder it is for his lungs to outgrow the harm being done to them by the mechanical ventilation.

Babies like Matthew are very hard to care for because their progress is so slow and they have so many other problems. He vomited intermittently, had hernias and gastrointestinal obstructions. All of these problems were related.

One autumn morning, nine weeks after his birth, Matthew was lying in an isolette adjacent to Angela Walker-Shaw, who had just begun to recover from her resection surgery. The doctors on morning rounds looked at her with approval, then turned glum as they shifted their attention to Matthew.

Matthew lay, froglike, on his belly, his head under an oxygen hood, his skin shriveled like a dried prune. He still weighed only 1005 grams (2 lb. 4 oz.), and he had not been gaining. Two walnut-sized hernias protruded from his groin. Hernias are not unusual in low-birth-weight babies. Their abdominal muscles are undeveloped and a lump of intestine sometimes pops out through a weak spot in the abdominal wall. It goes back in when the baby relaxes. But sometimes it gets caught. Then the baby becomes very agitated and is clearly in terrible pain. He vomits, his stomach bloats. Gas builds up, blocked by the hernia from escaping and preventing the hernia from receding. The belly distends, veins standing out as on a tight drum skin. Pressure builds against the diaphragm, impeding breathing further. This had repeatedly been Matthew's problem.

His nurse looked harried. The baby had been squirming in obviously extreme discomfort and setting off alarms on the monitors. Their sharp bleeps were just one more irritant. The nurse told the doctors that Matthew was "borderline." She said it was clear to her that he was in pain. But a resident replied that the baby would have to get stronger before a hernia operation could be attempted.

The team moved on. After receiving a dose of chloral hydrate, a hypnotic drug, Matthew calmed down. Then the respiratory therapist came with a nebulizer (atomizer), to try to give him some relief by blowing warm medicated mist under his hood in an effort to dilate the bronchial tubes, which were constricted because they had been traumatized by the endotracheal tube.

It is hard for the nurses to watch babies suffer like this without being able to do much for them. The doctors, who have many patients to care for, do not stay with one baby for eight hours at a time, day after day, watching him in pain and having to administer treatments that hurt still more. The nurse wished they could at least act on the hernias.

But by this time Matthew was in the bind that would keep him on the edge between death and recovery for a long, long time. "It's a catch-twenty-two," explained a neonatology fellow. "The hernias will be repaired when his lung disease gets better, but the lung disease won't get better until his nutrition is better, and his nutrition won't get better until the hernias are repaired."

The ray of hope rested on the possibility of helping the lungs along with a steroid treatment. During this time, Dr. Ronald Ariagno was conducting a double-blind study on the effectiveness of steroids in improving lung function of ventilator-dependent infants who are making no weaning progress at two weeks of age. The chance of such stalling is almost 70 percent after two weeks on the ventilator for infants of less than 1500 grams birth weight. Anyone as small as Matthew who is kept on the respirator more than two weeks has a good chance of getting stuck, that is, of developing chronic lung disease.

The subject of steroids is controversial. They have proved to be effective when administered before birth. The evidence on their use shortly after birth is still inconclusive. In the study, funded by the National Institutes of Health, Dr. Ariagno hoped to provide a firm answer. His own experience indicated that steroids were beneficial. Possible side effects, however, include alteration of immune defenses, hypertension, and growth delay.

Matthew was included in the study. Initial results were encouraging. Afterward, he managed to do without the ventilator for a few days. Then, however, he began to gasp for air again and was reintubated. The apparent slight progress encouraged physicians to try another course, then a third.

But the reports on Matthew continued to be depressing. At twelve weeks, the team at morning rounds heard, he had "not [been] doing well yesterday. Required oxygen. Was started on antibiotics. Too many things going wrong. Skin is really dry. X-ray still horrible."

At thirteen weeks: "Severely chronic lung disease. This kid's very sick."

At fourteen weeks: "Very much in a chronic pattern. Instabilities, secretion problems, weight down 90 grams today."

"His hernias are huge," remarked an intern.

"We usually don't touch them when a kid's that unstable," said the fellow.

"Can't he have a truss so they don't keep popping out?" asked the nurse.

"His buns are too small," replied the resident. "Matthew is still not gaining."

Because the hernias continued to obstruct his bowels, Matthew's belly continued to distend. He could not take in food, and he lost weight. Meanwhile, despite the three courses of steroids, the pulmonary condition was getting worse and worse till, by November, he was almost terminal.

By the end of November, everyone who knew and cared for Matthew was feeling very uncomfortable about his condition. His little body had been punctured with needles so many times that usable veins could no longer be found—not in wrists, ankles, scalp, or anywhere else. One night doctors worked for six hours trying to insert an IV. Finally, giving up, they had done a cut-down, risking more infection that would require still more medication. There was serious doubt now about whether Matthew had enough strength left ever to get off the ventilator. Was the treatment merely prolonging his inevitable demise? Was he being put through unnecessary suffering because the doctors had invested so much in him that they could not face letting him go?

The question came up at a time when the nursery staff was emotionally drained. It had been a hard month. Twice as many babies as usual had died, some of whom had been there a long time, and it was therefore harder for everyone to see them go. One of the fellows later said that Matthew was the next to be considered. Had the issue come up at a different time, with somebody else in charge, the next move might have been to take him off the ventilator and, if he did not make it—as was probable—allow him to expire. So thought this young physician. But others said no, none of the attendings would have gone that way yet, for there remained a flicker of hope. It hung on the question, Was Matthew still making an effort to breathe on his own, and, if so, was that effort in fact still moving some air? If the answer was negative, there clearly would be no point in continuing. If it was positive, a few more last-stand interventions would be justified to coax that flicker to grow into a steadier light.

The negative/positive dilemma could be resolved precisely in this nursery, for Dr. Ariagno had a piece of equipment, designed for his pulmonary function study with steroids, that could supply the information. A two-inch plastic tube with a stainless steel screen was attached to the baby's endotracheal tube. It measured the volume of air introduced by the ventilator or moved by the infant independently. It showed that Matthew was, indeed, still breathing effectively. That was the point at which Matthew began to acquire his reputation as a resilient little fellow, and people who, until then, had not particularly noticed him began to cheer for him. He lingered on into December, when Dr. Ariagno came on as the attending physician.

On his first morning back on service, Dr. Ariagno appeared in the nursery when the team was halfway through morning rounds. Usually, the attendings let the fellow take this first set of rounds, they themselves taking the afternoon ones. But Dr. Ariagno had come to get acquainted with the new team and the new set of patients.

The young doctors had already been through the intermediate nursery and were now grouped around a three-day-old thirty-four-weeker who had been transferred from Santa Cruz. Dr. Ariagno scanned the team: it seemed promising. The two interns would work well together: Melinda's outspokenness and wry humor balanced the shyness of Margie, whose voice was barely audible though her eyes seemed to miss nothing. The resident he knew as competent and quick; the fellow was a close associate. "Any students on board?" Dr. Ariagno asked. There were none. "Too bad." He was always pleased to have students along. They asked elemental questions and added a dimension he found creative and renewing.

The "on board" was in context. For the next weeks the team would be a tight crew, navigating in heavy waters. Last month, one of the house officers had caved in under the strain and had had to leave. Another collapsed in tears. It had been a tough month for all, as though a visitation of ill had come upon the place. This month could prove quite the opposite; one never knew. They might be able to send everyone home to grow up and be normal.

As the team continued to move from one little patient to another, discussing the day's plan and status for each one, the attending was briefed by his predecessor on the babies who would need his attention most urgently. Matthew Cordell's name topped the list.

The Cordell family seemed to be in a calamitous state. Part of the cause for its dissolution may have been the stress created by the baby's long hospitalization. Circumstances were unclear, but Sophie Cordell had been away for the past week and the couple's two other children were with relatives. Apparently the mother had felt she was being blamed for the infant's condition. She had returned, at the request of the staff, and had spent the preceding night in the parents' room.

Dr. Ariagno glanced toward Room One, where Sophie, a tall woman, sat straight-backed beside Matthew's crib, her legs crossed, swinging her right foot in a rhythm that betrayed her nervousness. He would confer with her and her husband after he had had a chance to evaluate Matthew who, according to reports, was still in a borderline state, as he had been three months earlier, when Dr. Ariagno had ended his last rotation.

The monthly shift of attendings is always a time of decision, some of the nurses have observed. Just before it happens, physicians sometimes take action on infants who have been lingering a long time. Nurses believe that aggressive treatment tends to be withdrawn more frequently toward the end of the month, though one of the attendings says this is anecdotal information that his own experience contradicts. In any event, the physician who is leaving knows that when his successor comes in, he might not do anything drastic for a while, wanting to reassess the situation. He is likely to put the baby through his own set of interventions, which the previous attending had not thought to try. Each of the physicians has a different approach, a different research interest, different strengths. If the departing attending feels that the case is hopeless, he might try to spare the baby that extra suffering.

But in situations like Matthew Cordell's, where the prognosis is not entirely clear to the attending, possible escalation of treatment may be postponed to allow the incoming doctor to proceed his own way. The rotation of attendings has the benefit of allowing long-term ICN residents to get the benefits of all three approaches. At the same time, it confuses the picture for parents, and fuzzes responsibility, so that sometimes a baby is continued to the point where, in the eyes of nurses and others, the treatment has begun to do harm rather than good.

A resident told Dr. Ariagno that the previous attending had "interpreted Matthew as salvageable."

"I think he is," the neonatologist said. "But it depends on whether he will get more lung damage before he starts improving." He knew, from the results of the pulmonary function study, that Matthew did not have much time left. He had to start getting well or he would exhaust his reserves and deteriorate beyond the reach of any further treatment.

Matthew lay on his side, at six months still smaller than most newborns. His breath squeaked like a rubber toy.

"Sounds like he's snoring," said Dr. Ariagno. "He has a leak around his tube and his lung is noncompliant." Scarred and thickened, the lungs had lost their resilience. The physician put the stethoscope on the baby's chest, holding a finger on the ventilator alarm to prevent it from going off. He felt the belly, determined that the liver was huge. He was tachypnic—he breathed very fast. The skin on his feet and hands was bluish.

Dr. Ariagno lifted one of Matthew's spindly arms and observed its lead-pipe rigidity. As he slowly attempted to flex it, however, it suddenly gave way at the elbow joint. This was characteristic of spastic muscles. "It could be that even if he was cured and survived his lung disease he would have cerebral palsy," Dr. Ariagno said. He decided to give a brief lunchtime talk to the team about survivors of chronic lung disease.

The rest of the morning moved at a rapid clip. Aside from being the first day of a new rotation, it was a typical day in the ICN. There was a transport to arrange, a delivery coming in. There were X-rays to look at. "Oh gosh!" Dr. Ariagno exclaimed in dismay, seeing Matthew's exploded belly projected on a screen. "Yeah," said the resident. "And he's got huge hernias that slide in and out and irritate the bowels. We used to call in the surgeons but we have given that up." (The surgeons were holding out for respiratory improvement.) And, as usual, there were people representing the developer of another new piece of equipment, hoping for a chance to try it out here. This time two salespersons presented instrumentation to measure fontanel or intracranial pressure, which might be elevated with hydrocephalus. Dr. Ariagno thought it worth a trial.

At noon he was in the conference room, slide projector ready. House staff came in, their sandwiches on paper plates. He began to talk about chronic lung disease and the way it acts on the lung, damaging normal lung architecture and limiting function. He explained how, after some weeks of ventilation, a premature infant's airway narrows, the lungs become stiff. Even with high-pressure air, some parts of the lung are not adequately ventilated. The baby remains hungry for air and gasps in an attempt to get more, but his exertions worsen the lung dysfunction, causing increased air hunger, increased effort and rapid breathing, a more rapid heart rate, and further exacerbation of the condition.

The attendings often used these noontime sessions to teach about the clinical problems of patients in the ICN. After this one, Dr. Ariagno had formulated his plan for Matthew: a fresh try at stabilizing his lungs with a combination of drugs that would open his airways, dry out his lungs, and with yet another course of steroids—his fourth—to try to improve his lung functon.

Many questions about the baby's status remained unanswered. Was Matthew intact in other ways? Would he be retarded? Would he have cerebral palsy? Trouble digesting? Those issues would have to wait until he was less critical and a bit older. One fact that contributed to the staff's eagerness to save him, however, was the EEG reading, which supported the view that his brain was still intact.

The conference over, the house staff scattered to perform their various duties. Dr. Ariagno stayed a few minutes longer to eat his tuna on rye. A research nurse stopped by for a chat with the doctor. He told her how a man had stopped him on the street the other day, saying, "You're Dr. Ariagno? You took care of my baby," and how he had steeled himself, not knowing what would come next. "Luckily," he said, "the baby is just fine." When asked why he pressed on with Matthew, given his bleak condition, he responded, "Human beings are very capable. To not even accept the challenge would be wrong. He's borderline. I'm not sure he will have cerebral palsy. He has a lot of problems, but they haven't all been active at the same time. I think he still has a chance."

At 1:00 P.M., returning to the nursery, the doctor found drastic changes in some of the babies. They were like mountain weather—you could not tell from one moment to the next what to expect from the borderline ones.

It was a normal day—one emergency after another. At 3:30 there was a breather, of sorts, as staff gathered in the conference room for the twice-a-month nursery management meeting, which provides a chance to bring up issues that are neglected during the hustle of daily work. Two attendings and several interns, residents, and nurses crowded into the small room.

One of the interns was depressed. "I haven't had a baby with a normal brain since I've been here," she complained. "Don't take it personally," Dr. Ariagno advised, smiling. Others, too, felt emotionally battered by the past few weeks.

"Best cure I can think of is to hold a routine baby and remember that these ICN infants are exceptions," he said. "There are a lot of very sick kids who got out without a scratch." But then he added, "Though I remember the name of every one who did not."

The day in the nursery ended for Dr. Ariagno with afternoon rounds followed by X-ray rounds. At 5:40 P.M., he checked the board behind the reception desk for transports and deliveries that were under way and decided that it looked like a quiet night. He would go down to the lab for a while to catch up on a little research and then head home for dinner. With luck, the evening would be his family's.

The doctors' day-to-day reality is their work within this particular context, which demands compliance with certain assumptions. It mandates efficiency, speed, attention to detail, and precision. Even for the most compassionate physicians, it does not allow for the slower rhythms and idiosyncratic expressions of parents who find they are primitives in this futuristic community, forced to deal for their children's lives with whatever resources they have.

Modern neonatology requires distancing; the human being craves connection. But the setting defines reality, and those who work here agree to accept it as the sane standard by which other realities are measured. One can only assume that the reality of the newborn is radically different from that of his medical caretakers. Nurses see themselves as spokespersons for the newborns' reality. In some ways, they feel as though they must defend the newborns from the physicians' painful intrusions. As Dr. Ariagno's day in the nursery ended, Matthew Cordell remained the recipient of technical and medical attention from an array of personnel. His nurse, while discussing her role as defender, said: "We feel that our job is to remind the doctors that the patients are babies and they hurt."

As if on cue, a senior resident approached and said she wanted to take a blood culture. This meant an arterial puncture, and the nurse knew it would hurt, from watching babies' reactions and hearing adults describe it as painful.

"Good luck," said the nurse. Staff had been trying to avoid sticking Matthew lately because his arteries were so sclerotic. "But could you wait till he gets his morphine?"

The resident agreed to that. The nurse waited until the sched-uled time, then inserted a morphine container into the baby's central line. The resident soon returned, carrying a high-inten-sity gooseneck lamp. She placed the light close to the baby's left heel, which became a translucent red. She felt for an artery. Mat-thew squirmed. He had been awakened, and he knew what was coming.

Before the resident had finished, however, an X-ray technician had come into the room and set up beside the adjacent baby. All the adults were asked to withdraw while he did his work. It took only a minute, but when it was over, the resident had gone. So Matthew had been awakened and disturbed for nothing. The nurse went to look for the resident and was told that she had gone to the delivery room. When the doctor finally returned forty min-utes after the morphine was given, the baby was again asleep, and the nurse asked the resident to wait again, until Matthew got his next dose two hours later. "You can see, it's hard for the babies to get their sleep," said the nurse.

It was two weeks before Christmas. Baby Matthew continued his struggle on the brink of existence, neither recovering nor ex-piring. The steroids seemed to help, but then he had an abdomi-nal distension episode, and all the support systems again had to be cranked up. Finally, toward the end of the month, Dr. Ariagno decided that the problem holding him back was the hernias. They would have to be repaired while he was on the respirator or he would exhaust his remaining reserves.

He put his plan before Dr. Sunshine and the surgeons, all of whom thought it was a poor idea and far too risky. They discussed it for a long time and in the end, the surgeons simply refused to perform the operation. But Dr. Ariagno was convinced he was on the right track. Either they did something about the hernias or they might as well pull the tubes. So he did something unusual but not unprecedented: he started looking for another surgeon who might see things his way and do the hernia repair. He also kept after the pediatric surgeons, who relented and scheduled surgery for Christmas Eve. The parents were called to a meeting.

Matthew's family was holding together as tenuously as the baby himself clung to life. The main glue that kept it together was Matthew's small, tortured self, the fulcrum of his parents' anxiety, yet the linchpin in their relationship. Indeed, one could make a good argument that Matthew had been born with a mission, so momentous was his role in this family's life.

The agony of the continuing uncertainty clawed at the fragile relationship Matthew Sr. and Sophie had reconstructed. But it also kept them together, for as long as their baby was in critical condition, everything else was pushed into the background.

Matthew Sr. was working forty-eight hours a week; Sophie had a full-time temporary job; and both of them took classes on Saturdays. They came to the hospital when they could—Sophie more often than her husband, who was afraid of becoming attached and then watching the baby die. Once, Sophie recalled, two weeks had gone by without her visiting. When she returned, she found that the baby had been moved to another location in the nursery and that his condition had changed. She vowed she would not let that much time pass again without her seeing him. Sophie worried about the future. "When he comes out of the hospital I'll have to give up my job. I like being out and around a lot of people. Staying home—I can do it, but . . ." A trap seemed to be closing in on her.

Meanwhile, her in-laws viewed her with suspicion, wondering if all this was, somehow, her fault. Their son told them he did not want to hear such suggestions. But they stuck in his mind nevertheless and added to the tension between him and his wife. "Sometimes I think it was all a big mistake," Matthew said at one point. "That I should have let her stay in the navy and not tried to get her back. If the baby dies, that's it. That will be the last mistake we ever make together."

So Matthew Jr., the catalyst for his parents' reunion, was the focal point of their distress. He was, of course, only a baby, barely a baby, and innocent of any contrivance. Unless, of course, one held to the notion—a tenet of some faiths—that we choose where and how we are born. If that is so, then Matthew had chosen a hard life indeed.

Several times he came within breaths of expiring. The doctors would call in his parents for conferences and, as gently as they could, convey the message that he would probably not live. They would brace themselves. But then he would pull through again.

Once they were called in for good news: he was off the ventilator. He was doing better. But as they were leaving the parents' conference room, they saw that nurses and interns had crowded around their baby and were working on him. He had had a relapse. He was going back on the ventilator.

The enormous hospital costs, which soon were higher than what the parents could expect to earn in a lifetime, were a worry to Matthew Sr. for some time. He felt that the military should cover them, for Sophie was in the reserves. She had done what she had been told to do: sought care in the nearest hospital during the pregnancy, gone to the nearest military hospital when labor started, then to a community hospital, from where she was sent to Stanford. However, the navy authorities found a clause— "which we had never seen and never signed," said Matthew—that excluded coverage in cases where care was given in a civilian hospital. He made so many phone calls trying to straighten out the situation that his supervisor reprimanded him and he feared for his job. Benefits of the job included an excellent health plan, but it appeared that the baby had been born two days too soon to qualify.

The skilled and helpful patient representative at the medical center offered to help the Cordells apply for the state's MediCal coverage and said that the California Children's Services, a state program for disabled children, would also be able to meet some of the expense. But for Matthew it was a matter of principle. "Why should society pay for this when it's the military's responsibility?" he argued. Eventually, however, he gave in and applied for federal and state aid. Shortly thereafter, his employer found that Matthew Sr.'s health plan covered the baby after all. So the bill was taken care of, easing the Cordells' minds a little, but not much. In a way, the hospital costs had been, beyond a certain point, like the national debt—unreal.

In their personal economics, the big item was the house, which they had bought in October, at about the time Matthew, Jr. had originally been expected, in a subdivision of San Jose. The payments stretched their budget to the limit and required more than Matthew's salary, at least for a while. Sophie would have to quit her job if the baby came home. How they could afford that was unclear, for even with both of them earning money, at times they were compelled to give up their telephone because they could not pay the bill.

They had already given up their Saturday classes so they could visit the hospital, and they had sent Sophie's older son to his grandfather in Texas, to spare him the anxiety they were experiencing. Their two-year-old daughter was showing the effects of the tension, becoming demanding, and they were impatient with her. Everything was undone and uncertain.

The day before the scheduled hernia operation, Sophie remarked, "I feel like we're between a rock and a hard place. I want him to live, but I don't want him to be retarded. There is just that one guarantee I wish they could give me, that he won't be retarded. But I know they can't. Right now they can't even say if he will live. In five months he has not progressed that much."

She felt a distance between herself and this baby that she had not felt with her other two children. This one had been so inaccessible, and her role with him had been so odd. "It was two months before we could hold him," she said. "Now, when we go to see him, it's just visiting. You go visit an hour, then you leave him. It's a bond, but not a strong bond. Not like with her," she said, meaning her older child, "where you take her to a baby-sitter and you know you're going to pick her up again later in the day. Here it's like, you can go anytime, but you know he's not going to come home. His home is at the hospital."

Three days after Christmas, Dr. Ariagno greeted his team at afternoon rounds by announcing, "Well, everyone is either smaller or not any better." He was smiling as he said it, so he got some laughs in response. The year was ending, and so was his month on duty in the nursery. The attendings often seem more cheerful and light-spirited as their rotations wind toward their conclusion.

On this day, however, the nursery was jammed with forty patients—capacity. Among the new ones was a set of healthy triplets born somewhat prematurely to a couple who already had eight children between them, from previous marriages, but had wanted to have one together so badly that they had sought in vitro fertilization and been thrice lucky. The mother, who was thirty-six, had first tried to have a tubal ligation reversed. When this did not work, the couple had tried one of the new, expensive, and awkward procedures for conception that are available to people who cannot manage impregnation the usual way. So here were these babies, lying on their little beds, in their little green knit caps, emissaries of the future reaching into the nursery. Their pictures were on the front pages of several local papers with headlines: FIRST BAY AREA IN VITRO TRIPLETS.

Matthew, in Room One, was definitely better. The hernia operation had been followed by a rapid improvement in ventilation. The respirator settings were turned down. Carbon dioxide (CO_2) retention was far lower than it had been earlier. Matthew was on total parenteral nutrition, on the intravenous formula, and because he had been tolerating his feeds, would soon be weaned from TPN and shifted to nasal gavage feedings. Dr. Ariagno envisioned a two-week course. After that, Matthew could probably begin to nipple and, given his age, go on solid baby foods. Meanwhile, the improvement in his breathing indicated his readiness to be weaned from the ventilator.

"Glorious," said one of the interns.

"Amazing," said Dr. Ariagno. He pulled back the baby's blanket and looked at Matthew's back, which was moving rhythmically, without much collapse of the chest being evident. That meant that Matthew was tolerating the lower ventilator settings and doing a significant amount himself. "Look at the way he's breathing," said the doctor, with real joy in his voice. "And his belly has stayed soft." He saw his judgment as vindicated: the removal of the hernia problem had allowed the baby to tolerate feedings and to begin to improve in breathing.

The surgeons, to be sure, had their own interpretation. They argued that the factor causing trouble had not been the hernias, it had been the morphine that Matthew had been receiving for so long. Morphine slows down the metabolism, they contended, and therefore interfered with the baby's digestive system. However, the infant was given morphine after the surgery but suffered no more bowel distension.

Dr. Ariagno felt Matthew's belly, then went to the sink in the center of the room to scrub down with Betadine before proceeding to the next baby. As he did so he gave instructions to the team about the next step. Matthew was to be put on continuous positive airway pressure (CPAP) the following day. Pressurized air would be delivered to him in a continuous flow, through a face mask, to keep his airways open as he increased his own effort to breathe. If he showed sufficient breathing activity with that, the endotracheal tube would be removed.

To make sure that the transition from respirator to CPAP was as smooth as possible, Dr. Ariagno asked that the fellow insert the nasal gastric (NG) feeding tube that night, so any upset it might cause could be dealt with while Matthew was still on the ventilator.

Matthew, then, was doing well—for him. However, his history must be borne in mind: repeated improvement, followed by extubation, followed by what the Stanford doctors call an acute crash. Though one cause for those crashes had been removed, he was so frail that he was vulnerable to many things, especially the viruses and bacteria that are never—despite the staff's most valiant efforts—eliminated from the nursery. He had repeatedly upset the physicians' plans for him and indeed, four days after his hernia repair, did so once more.

The team had not gone far into the main nursery when Matthew's nurse came after Dr. Ariagno: Matthew had extubated himself. His hands had not been pinned down to the mattress, as they often were to prevent just that from happening.

"All right," said Dr. Ariagno, "let's do now what we planned to do tomorrow. Put him on mask CPAP right now. First put in the NG tube, then give him some Vaponefrin [a medicated mist that reduces vocal cord swelling], then put on the mask."

The fellow and two nurses peeled off from the rounds to carry out these instructions. What they had to do is not something anyone enjoys, most particularly not Matthew, who struggled against his constraints and his handlers, even though he was on two tranquilizers, Valium and phenobarbitol.

The nurses sat him up. One nurse hand-bagged him as the other jammed in the NG tube. "Come on, Matthew, swallow the tube," she urged. He gagged. He flailed with his arms, the right splinted and bandaged to provide a platform for that hard-to-insert IV. He gargled, arched, struggled. His hands reached up, as though for help. "I think I don't like this assignment anymore," said one of the nurses. She had taken on Matthew today because she thought he was easy.

"He looks bluish," said the fellow. "Let's give him some more O's." He turned up the oxygen in the mix being pumped into the baby's lungs. Meanwhile, the nurses slipped the white lacy net over the baby's face and attached the rubber face mask, which connects to the ventilator circuit to provide constant airway pressure to keep the lungs open.

The team, meanwhile, had proceeded down the row of babies next to the window of the main room. They were looking at the in vitro triplets, who were fine and due to go home very soon. The attending suggested that the young doctors might take a look at a recent issue of *Time*, which featured an article listing twelve new artificial ways to conceive babies. Someone said he had heard that other mammals are being tried out as surrogates and—though this was fantasy—in the ICN it did not really sound like that farfetched an idea.

At this point Matthew's nurse reappeared with a yellow slip of paper showing the results of a blood gas test: the baby was again retaining CO_2. This meant he would again be air-hungry and require more mechanical assistance. So Dr. Ariagno left the team and returned to the distressed baby. It was 5:22 P.M. when he took over the bagging.

"He's wild," said Matthew's nurse. "I've given him Valium." His other drugs at the moment were Decadron, Lasix, and antibiotics.

"Want to try some Bronkosol, too?" asked Dr. Ariagno. The nurse responded by attaching the nebulizer to the tube on the bag. The mix Matthew received was now moist and medicated.

"He's very squeaky at the moment," said Dr. Ariagno. "This is a baby that needs to calm down. It's really not that bad, even if he wasn't ready for extubation."

The baby was wheezing and his breath again squeaked like a rubber toy. Beyond the reach of his tortured eyes, a bright picture of a snowman, done by a child, hung above his crib, with the message "Happy Five Months."

Dr. Ariagno was trying to determine whether the current problem was fluid in the lungs, which were "like a leaky roof," or a constriction of the airway leading to them. Babies who are on a ventilator for a long time, who have a tube down their throat for months, develop a kind of scar tissue below their vocal cords, which, when they are upset, leads to collapse of the airways due to an extreme effort across the partial obstruction. He found out by putting the endotracheal tube back; immediately the breathing improved. This meant that there was an obstruction.

"His cords are terrible," he said to the nurse. "He may need bronchoscopy and surgical treatment" (to remove the damaged tissue in the airway). Some ventilator-dependent babies may require several treatments. "We'll see what happens tomorrow."

The first days of 1985 saw Matthew off the ventilator, under a plastic tent, breathing on his own with the help of supplemental oxygen administered through a nasal cannula, a tube that ran under his nostril. For the first time he could be heard crying. It was not a cry, really, but a croak, like that of a weak frog. But a few days later it was in a stronger voice, with more tone. A respiratory therapist who listened to his lungs heard a rustling, as of paper being crinkled—the sound of fluids and secretions.

In mid-January, Matthew had been stable long enough to allow tests of his general condition. His brain was intact, as far as could be determined. There was no hydrocephalus. The EEG was "fairly normal," according to one of the physicians. "Of course, he is enormously delayed developmentally because he has been so sick," he added. "A seven-month-old would at least coo, would roll over and sit up and crawl. He can't do these things. His neurological development is severely impaired. He is at risk for CP. It will be years before his lungs get back to normal—if they ever do. And I always feel very nebulous about the developing personalities of these very small and sick babies. All of us have a great deal of difficulty with babies like this. But perhaps because I have seen a large number of them grow up to be functional toddlers, I think it is very worthwhile to take care of them."

Was there ever a time when he could have been allowed to expire? he was asked.

He saw none. "If he had not been breathing at all, if the ventilator had been doing everything for him at six months, we would have had a different philosophy. But the pulmonary function test given then showed that he was able to ventilate, so he had a chance. Now, if he gets sick again, someone will have to decide whether to intubate him again. If his lung disease improves, they will. If it progresses, if there is evidence of heart failure, they probably would not. Compassion would indicate, in the case of a very sick baby that is dying anyway, that he should die in his mother's arms rather than connected to a lot of tubes."

But the next time Matthew began gasping and threatened to die without ventilator support, he was reintubated immediately, with no deliberations. His crisis was brought on, it appeared, by being moved to another location, from the quieter Room One to the main nursery.

"I stuck in an ET tube and an IV, and he's a lot better now," said Dr. Will Salomon, who came to Matthew's rescue.

The attending during January was filling in for a regular staff member who was on sabbatical. At the end of his time, he said he was "depressed about this baby's future, but I'm not going to make any major moves because there are a lot of people here who have devoted much more time and thought to him. I think the issue is going to get forced sometime in the next two weeks."

By this time Matthew was an important member of the ICN family, someone many people cared about and had invested in. He was the senior citizen of the nursery. The bill for his care was up to $420,000. But the weeks passed, the next attending was again about to go off service, and—at seven months now—Matthew was still borderline.

As sometimes happens in such cases, the primary nurses asked for a meeting. It seemed to those who knew Matthew best that the nursery may have done as much as it could for him. So one afternoon, the people who had been most intimately involved with the Cordells gathered in the little conference room. The group included a fellow, an intern, a physical therapist, two of his three primary nurses, Amy Goodwin and Mae Adair, and the discharge coordinator, Kathy Petersen. Notably absent was the attending physician. He was en route from Monterey, said the fellow.

One of the nurses observed, with a slight edge in her voice, that "this has been scheduled for a long time."

"Don't ask me. I just work here," responded the fellow.

Amy began the discussion, coming right to the point. As far as she could see, nothing much was happening with Matthew. "What is your criterion for him? What is expected before he can go home?"

The fellow said that the attending had wanted it conveyed that two weeks of weight gain without problems would be required before the baby could go home, even if skilled nursing care were sent along. "Do you think neonatal nurses—if he were home—could handle what he has gone through the last couple of nights?" he asked.

Matthew had been extremely agitated, and had repeatedly worked himself up into an extraordinary hunger for air.

"Emotionally and developmentally, he's going down the tubes," said Amy.

"He looks identical to Angela," put in the physical therapist. "He gets bug-eyed like she did, he startles easily. A lot of noises set him off. The alarms make him jump. So does the garbage can lid."

Indeed, the intern had also observed the similarity with the Walker-Shaw baby. She had been startled to see it, coming back on service after an absence of seven months. Matthew had been arching his back more and more, the way Angela had. He had begun to throw up his food, just as Angela had, for reasons his caretakers thought were psychological. And he was again failing to gain weight.

"He's not as bad as Angela yet, but he's getting there," said Mae. "He's not reaching for toys, not playing."

"The next step," said the PT, "is nipple refusal. It took Angela two weeks to get to that after she started to withdraw and became bug-eyed."

Matthew's caretakers all agreed that the ICN environment did not seem to be doing him much good now and was probably doing harm. He had to get out of it. But how?

"The family is having a lot of troubles. They are attached to Matthew, but they are a bit unrealistic. They have never spent an entire day with him," said Kathy. "The parents keep asking us to give them a date. We've dragged them in repeatedly to tell them 'your kid is going to die.'"

"We've done that to plenty of parents," responded the fellow. "The message is not really as important as the underlying commitment to the kid. You have Veronica Petras at the other extreme."

There was judgment in the physician's words, the implication being that perhaps these parents did not care enough. Some young doctors tend to be short on the kind of life experience that makes for empathy. There were vast differences between the Cordells and the Petras family. Veronica's parents were affluent. They also wanted a baby desperately and had gone to great lengths to conceive. The Cordells, on the other hand, were among the many families who just barely manage to hang on to the bottom edge of middle-class life, aware that the chasm of poverty is never far from the doorstep. They were not ready for Matthew when he came. They were trying, they were loving, and they could not be fairly compared with the Petrases. The nurses knew this. So Amy spoke up for the Cordells. "They are scared to death to bring him home."

Kathy jumped in with support. "I'm overwhelmed at how much the parents have to learn to take him home. What if they can't?" she posited, the realist ready to examine the options. "They may need medical foster care."

"If they can't handle it, it's gonna be death for the kid if they take him home," said the fellow. "We need a contingency plan."

Kathy, realizing from previous experience that parents feel guilty and torn at the thought of such a proposal, said, "Tell them it's okay. It's okay if you feel overwhelmed. But you have to let us know. With one family that had a baby go home with a tracheostomy, it was two weeks before they finally said they couldn't do it."

It was clear to all that the parents somehow had to confront their options and that this could best be done if they learned what taking Matthew home would mean. The only way to learn that was by spending time caring for him in the ICN.

"We'd do the family a big favor by forcing them to come in, forcing them to face their own limitations," said the fellow.

"Dad has to travel to LA three, four days at a time. He's in the reserves and has to report this weekend," said a nurse.

"Will Mom have to quit work for a few weeks?" asked Amy.

"The job she has now is temporary, but it's turning into a permanent position," said Kathy. "Her job is very important to her."

"She's the kind of person who can't face being home twenty-four hours a day," added a nurse.

"If we tell her that he's going home March 28, could she get four or five days off?" someone asked.

"A week," said Kathy.

In the end the group agreed that the nurses would work out a schedule for the parents, one that would require each of them to spend a minimum of four hours at a time every two days during the last week of Matthew's stay, taking care of him. They knew that their target date for discharge might require revision, but it was at least something to work toward.

That long-range issue settled, they turned toward the immediate problem of improving life for Matthew right then. The PT drew on the Angela Walker-Shaw experience: "Consistency of care will be most important. He's bonded to certain people. And he will need a quieter environment, so he won't get into those agitated states."

"What triggers his episodes?" asked the fellow.

"As soon as Matthew wets his diaper he wakes and starts screaming. Even if it's just a little bit," Mae said she'd found. "You've got to get to him right away or he escalates. I've also seen him go crazy when he's left in the swing too long in one position."

The nurses shared practical suggestions for helping the baby to cope: Minimize intrusions. Maybe let him go for a five-hour stretch without bothering him with anything, so he can sleep. Maybe move him to the window, to the spot where Angela was during the last part of her stay, so he would not be between two beeping monitors. Maybe not take his vital signs every two hours, maybe skip a feeding, so he gets a chance to sleep longer. "If there is some consistency in his life, perhaps he'll feel he has some control," said the PT.

These simple, commonsense measures would, ideally, be part of normal nursery care. But they are often omitted amid the emergencies, the many overlapping daily routines involving so many people, and the preeminence of focus on the acute care technology and medical measures.

But beyond the family situation and the steps to improve Matthew's circumstances, another unspoken question had been waiting. It had been there, looming as the invisible but terribly palpable shadow beside his crib during all the months of his struggle. Amy asked it: "If he needed to be intubated again—would we?"

The answer came with no hesitation from the fellow. "I think so. Doing it would just buy you time to make the right decision for him. If it comes down to that, I wouldn't want people to make the decision in the middle of the night. I'd like to do it in the light of day. If he got acute sepsis or something, of course, intubation would make no difference."

So there it was again. At birth, all babies are routinely resuscitated, no matter what their condition, "to buy time" for the right decision. Later, the simple fact that they are alive seems to call for measures to keep on, despite the mounting cost in suffering. Because Matthew had been so sick for so long, moments of decision had presented themselves—or could have—more than once. Always, for one reason or another, the choice had been to take just one more step and think about the situation later. And so he had lingered—improving slightly, then falling ill once more because he had no resiliency and any little infection or imbalance pushed him off the frail stability his organism now and then established. Again his growth would stop, again someone would say, "Well, he did better than we had expected so he must have something going." And they would go on. Would Matthew be one of those babies who go home, finally, only to die there?

Mae moved in on the shadow. "The father asked, 'Will he do this at home?'"

"He might. He might die at home." The fellow heard the unspoken question.

The meeting ended, and the fellow left to talk with another parent. The women continued to discuss Matthew's behavior, his feeding, his future. They referred repeatedly to their experience with Angela, and that reminded them of one big difference: unlike Matthew, she had had the benefit of daily visits from her parents and often from her grandmother.

"It would be nice if somebody would sit with their two-year-old sometimes, so they could come in for longer," said one of the nurses.

"I asked Sophie if she had any friends here, and she said she doesn't," the other one said.

"I could sit Sunday . . ." said the PT, tentatively. The nurses objected immediately; they did not think it was a good idea. But the suggestion showed the depth of these staffers' involvement with Matthew.

At this point, the attending finally arrived. He poured himself a cup of coffee and turned toward the women. They ignored him and continued talking. He sat down at the head of the table, in the chair vacated a few minutes earlier by his fellow, and seized the next pause to say "I'm sorry I'm late. There was a three-car wreck on Seventeen and traffic was backed up for forty-five minutes." If not for that, he would have arrived exactly on time—three minutes early, in fact.

Nobody asked about the accident, but Amy turned to him for a prognosis on Matthew.

"Medically it's only a week he's been better," the neonatalogist said. "If he has one to three weeks of steady growth we can consider his going home." Then he added, illuminating the classic difference in perspective between doctors and nurses, "He's walking the narrowest possible path. I confronted him several times with death and he just gets mad at me and goes on."

It was an affectionate remark and it was respectful of the baby as a person. It also suggested that for this tall, handsome, and aloof doctor, the practice of medicine was not unlike war. He was a warrior against death, proud and compassionate and protected by armor, who recognizes courage when he sees it in the troops and gallantly gives it its due.

It was a remark that grew out of Matthew's rising reputation as a baby who would not give up, and the kind of remark that fed that image of him.

But this attending was a father as well, and he had a capacity for deep empathy. He was not oblivious to the babies' suffering. "My fear is, regarding his going home, that the first cold he gets he goes into heart failure," he said. "Or, if he loses any more alveoli . . . On the other hand, he'll have a shot. Staying here, he can get nastier things."

Later, outside the meeting, he explained the "confronted him with death" remark. "He's a tough little kid. Some people, you say they can't make it and they'll spit in your face. When there is no hope except through a tiny chink, they will go for it." His chances were not too good, with lungs so very damaged, there was always the possibility of heart failure because the right side of the heart had to work harder to get oxygen. Chronic ventilator babies have that problem. Most grow out of it. But the physician knew that Matthew was "the kind of kid who can develop severe right heart failure and slide right off."

The parents should be told, he said, that if they decide they cannot take care of him and that he needs medical foster care, "that does not mean that they have to give him up. If he continues to develop and grow, they can take him home. It just means that he does not have to live in the hospital. What he really needs is a nurse twenty-four hours a day."

As everyone began leaving the room, the attending again brought up the cause of his lateness, "It was quite something, actually—a Jaguar, a truck, and an old car with Mexican-American families. I thought I might be called in to be a Good Samaritan, but I looked and the children were all right." Nobody seemed curious to know more. Dramas are a dime a dozen here.

The meeting over, Amy and Mae went into the nursery, one to visit the subject of their discussion for a few moments, the other to take over his care. They looked silently at the baby for a moment. "He'll probably be the most difficult baby we ever send home," said Mae. Matthew began to cry. It was a strange, strangled sound, more like a chicken's than a human baby's. Amy patted his bottom. The crying and squirming did not stop. So she picked him up slowly, put him on her lap and patted his back. She herself had asthma, so she empathized very personally with Matthew's struggle to breathe. Like Mae, she had wished that his struggle could end. This was just too much for a baby to suffer. And if, after all this, he should live, what kind of life could he have, being so frail? Personally, and professionally, she felt discouraged. "This baby is the sum total of the past seven months of my work," she said, pausing in her back-patting for a moment to spread her hands. "To whose benefit has it all been?"

Before a week was out, the March 28 discharge date had come to appear overoptimistic. Shortly after the meeting about his future, Matthew developed something that was either, as one of the nurses said, bacterial pneumonia or, as one of the fellows said, just a cold. In his condition, the diagnosis did not really make much difference, for either was enough to send him into a downward slide again. He lost weight, had to go on a higher dosage of oxygen, and was put on intravenous hyperalimentation.

On February 27, Mae's day off, another nurse was taking care of him. She had been assigned to him occasionally, probably because she had considerable experience with chronic babies, she thought. In fact, she had been the primary nurse two years ago for a child who died at five and a half months, and whose condition had been similar to Matthew's.

Matthew had been moved to Angela Walker-Shaw's old place, the spot by the window, and a sign at the end of the bed asked that people not intrude on him unless absolutely necessary because he was suffering from "overstimulation." A blanket covered the top of the crib when he slept. But he was still trying to withdraw, arching way back, refusing to look at anyone directly. The nurse had seen this in other chronic infants. "They look like they are trying to get away," she said. "He's different with his parents," she added. "He does things for them he won't do for anyone else—as was also true with Angela. He looks at them steadily, without the scary bug eyes. Every time I've seen him with his parents he has been calm, quiet, and awake. He sits in a position that he usually finds uncomfortable, on the lap, and he makes clear eye contact. When I have him he fusses. I have to feed him belly-down on my lap. In the normal infant position, in my arms, he wiggles and fusses. That's what happens with these babies. If they are not too far gone and improve physically they eventually start rolling forward into the normal newborn position. But they have been on their bellies for so long."

She spoke softly, for Matthew was asleep on his belly with his diapered bottom pulled up, a little mound above his scrawny body with the elongated, flattened preemie head. But at this point two nurses, having business with her, came by, and their voices were a little louder. After they left, a respiratory therapist arrived and began to adjust Matthew's life-support equipment. The neighboring baby's monitor began to beep, as usual, because something needed adjusting, not because there was any need for alarm. Matthew awoke with a strange chicken cry. The nurse picked him up, the lines trailing behind him.

It was noisy here, even though Room One had been designated the quiet room after the trouble with Angela. "We do things with the babies we would never do with adult patients," one of the nurses reflected one day. "We forget. We talk across the incubators, for instance."

It was also noisy inside the incubators. "Sometimes, when you put your stethoscope on a baby's chest, all you hear is the hum of the isolette," Matthew's nurse said. She lowered the infant into the swing beside his crib and cranked up its mechanism, producing a loud, harsh sound of metal on metal. The baby was in the seat, an IV hanging from the top of his head, his arms extended rigidly, his back arched. His eyes were full of terror, darting around, focusing on nothing. He was a trapped creature, desperate to escape.

A few days later, Matthew, very sick, was transferred into isolation, a little room at the end of the main nursery, where the lights could be dimmed and the door shut, and only those who had business entered. The nurses thought he liked it better there. He rallied enough to return to Room One. The little room could not be his for long, anyway, because it was used for minor surgery and for infants who were being watched for possible infections, such as herpes, that were not otherwise present in the nursery.

As March rolled toward its end, the parents were once again called in, to discuss plans for going home. Matthew Sr. told the staff that he was willing to work two jobs so that Sophie could stay home and give the baby the care he required. She, however, turned gray at his words, so that Kathy Petersen was prompted to say to him, "Has it occurred to you, Matthew, that maybe Sophie works because she wants to, not because you need the money?" Medical foster care was mentioned, and also the possibility that Matthew's insurance policy would cover some home nursing care for a while. But when the meeting ended, staff members were left with the uneasy feeling that the conflicts that had once driven this couple to separate may have remained, having been postponed only by the eight-month-long ICN tenure of their baby. Could they stand the added burden of the homecoming of this very difficult, complicated baby?

Finally a day came when the doctors told the parents that little Matthew was ready to go home, on oxygen support. The parents were to come in to learn the details of the baby's care. The discharge was to take place within days, as soon as all arrangements were made.

On Friday, March 27, both parents arrived. This time, they had managed to leave their two-year-old daughter with a sitter, so that they could give their full attention to Matthew. They changed his diapers, played with him. Nurse Amy moved away, to allow them to feel more comfortable. They had made an appointment to see a public health nurse the following week, and to meet with a private physician. Dr. Sunshine talked with them about caring for the baby on oxygen at home. They left while Amy was still on duty.

When she went off shift she noticed that Matthew did not look good. He had been fussy all day. His tummy was bloated once again, and his breathing labored. "I knew he was looking bad, but he had done this so many times I thought he might be needing another septic workup, that he would have to go through that again," she later said. "I hoped not, because I remembered the time when we spent two and a half hours trying to start an IV and he gave me a look that said, 'Why are you doing this to me?' I couldn't bear it."

Matthew was now so old that he was undeniably a person. His needs were more varied than those of other babies in the nursery. He was awake for long periods of time and he needed to be played with. Often, he was playful during his meals, so that his feedings took as long as an hour and a half. He was aware of people and events around him. Some of his caretakers believed that he knew a great deal. Because he had developed his own habits and idiosyncracies, people who did not know him found him difficult to care for, while those who knew him well were becoming increasingly involved. Dr. Salomon, for instance, had discovered that if Matthew was cranky and he put his hand into his, the baby would calm down immediately. He was moved by Matthew's powerful direct gaze and found it increasingly difficult to do painful procedures with him.

It was definitely time for this baby to leave the ICN for a quieter, more peaceful, and less pain-ridden place. Now, as she watched the baby go into another one of his downs, Amy feared another delay in his scheduled departure. But she knew that the doctors were running out of ideas for helping Matthew. She had over-heard one of them say, just that day, that he was "a medical fail-ure." That had angered her: it was such an inhuman concept, applied to this child. As Amy left, she felt very downhearted, and once outside, she was glad to take a deep breath of the cold winter air and let the sound of the wind in the trees sweep through her mind.

By 3:15 P.M. Matthew's tummy was huge and the baby was gasping. The swing-shift nurse aspirated his stomach and brought up 70 cc of food and digestive juices. His belly now was flat but he was not better. The gastrointestinal system was down. The respiratory system was going down. Matthew was retracting, his chest was caving in with each hard-fought breath. How long could his heart continue to sustain such effort? She put a mask over his head and turned on the oxygen. She also gave him Lasix, for he had not urinated since late morning. But it produced no effect. The kidneys seemed to have stopped functioning.

Realizing that Matthew was heading for a full-blown code, with both respiratory and cardiac arrest, the nurse searched the baby's head for a vein that might take the inevitable new IV he required. She found none. The veins were simply gone. Another cut-down and deep line to the heart would be necessary. She called the pharmacist and prepared the drugs that would be required for the resuscitation.

But this time a hand of mercy reached out to stop the rescue machine. Dr. Sunshine was on duty. Perhaps this made a differ-ence, perhaps not. Perhaps anyone in charge at this moment would have done the same thing. But ICN staffers have observed that each of the senior physicians comes to the final decision point by his own personal route. One will watch a situation de-velop, say nothing for a long time, then decide that the moment has come when hope has vanished and it is time to release the baby from suffering. He is then likely to withdraw aggressive measures, consulting with colleagues but shouldering the re-sponsibility. Another, whose approach is more intellectual, some-times prepares for a decision by discussing the baby's problem, more or less in the abstract, during a midday lecture for house staff. "We know he is machinating on something when he sched-ules one of these," said a resident.

A third physician operates in a manner that is midway between the other two. He is a strong advocate for opening the process of decision making. Whenever possible, most prefer a group process of some sort and tend to resuscitate babies at least until such time as they can get a consensus. They all prefer to make their important decisions at bedside, after having consulted with nurses, social workers, other caregivers, and parents. If no consensus is reached, all will sometimes call an ethics committee meeting. But each must sometimes respond to a crisis without having time to think or plan, whether he is dealing with a newly arrived infant or a child who has been in the nursery for a long time.

Dr. Sunshine, the eldest and most experienced of the Stanford neonatologists, had the reputation of being most intuitive and most willing to make an irrevocable decision on his own. For this he was admired by many who knew him. They saw personal risks in his style, in light of the prevailing legal and political climate. But they trusted his judgment.

Alerted by Matthew's nurse to the baby's sudden collapse—his acute crash, in nursery language—Dr. Sunshine immediately saw that the child was exhausted and had no more strength for struggling. He consulted with Dr. Ariagno, who had been most involved with this patient and knew him better than he did. Dr. Ariagno agreed that it would be inhumane to escalate treatment. Heroic measures would be futile because Matthew no longer had the capacity for recovery. His entire system was breaking down. A call to the parents was placed.

In other hospitals, other physicians might have decided otherwise, for a variety of reasons. They might have succeeded in extending Matthew's misery a little longer. But the people who knew Matthew best agreed that nothing could be done to save him. "We all knew," Dr. Sunshine would reflect later, "that all we had done was to prolong this baby's dying."

At 5:30 P.M., Matthew's gasping was even more desperate. He was working himself up into the state of anxiety that would require ever more oxygen as breathing became less and less effective. He was, however, already receiving 100 percent oxygen.

At 5:45 P.M., his heart rate slowed and became irregular. The nurse bagged him. At 6:15 P.M., she put him under a Plexiglass hood to maximize his oxygen intake while she continued to bag him. Matthew's caretakers were trying to keep him until his parents could come to say good-bye. It took a while before the father was located at work and asked to come in because the baby was in critical condition. How often had he heard that message? Each time before this, Matthew had recovered.

The nurses kept bagging for another half hour. But it was no use. At 6:45 P.M. it was over. Matthew's heart stopped.

Someone had called Amy and Kathy Petersen at their homes and they had hurried back. By the time the Cordells arrived, knowing only that Matthew was in danger, Amy was holding his tightly wrapped body, free at last of tubes and needles and probes and of pain. She held him very close, saying good-bye. He was so light. Despite all their efforts, he had never reached five pounds.

The parents, still unaware, went into the scrub room, preparing to enter the nursery. Suddenly there was panic among the staff: Where was Dr. Sunshine? The other doctors were in the delivery room. Who was to stop the parents from reaching the bedside without having been told?

Dr. Sunshine appeared as Matthew and Sophie were putting on the hospital gowns before leaving the scrub room. He walked toward them. A moment later, a single piercing wail came from both parents. It ran the length of the main nursery and beyond. It broke the rules.

The initial shock over, Matthew Cordell grew angry. Why couldn't they bring his son back this time when they had done it so many times before? Why had they compelled him to come here, made him care, then betrayed him? They had forced him to know and love this child, then had allowed the child to die.

Kathy Petersen talked with both parents. She explained that "Matthew put up such a fight that we fought with him," and that "he decided that he did not want to live anymore."

The father was incredulous and also awed at the suggestion that a baby could decide whether to live or die. "A baby? I never knew that. . . ." Yet that idea did not really explain anything. It merely opened many new questions.

The Cordells did not hurry away. There was no other place for them to go at that moment, for they were with the only people who had known and cared for their son during his entire life, who shared their grief. They stayed to give Matthew his last bath and to wrap him one last time. Then they went home.

"We're going to need to stay in touch," said one of the staff.

Amy, Kathy, and others stayed on because they needed to talk. "He was sort of family," Kathy said later. "It was hard to lose him. There was something about his spirit that said, 'Nobody will make decisions for me.' He had a powerful presence. He had a powerful gaze. I wonder why he didn't check out earlier. He had so many opportunities. My perspective on these babies is that they make up their own minds," she continued. "You can do everything you want, but it is still the baby who decides. Matthew was born into a system where the technology could take care of him. Given that system, he chose his fate. Because when we said he was going to die he didn't, and when we said he would go home, he died."

"Everyone really wanted him to make it," reflected Dr. Salomon. "And sometimes that got in the way. Once, we got fooled about his weight. He was gaining, but it was because he was retaining fluid. His real weight was actually going down. But we wanted so much to think that he had made the transition from being real sick to being a growing kid that we got the wrong interpretation. Then he crashed. I can't believe how you can have this incredible attachment to an eight-month-old preemie."

"I don't think it was a mistake to try," said another doctor. "For him it was right, to give him the maximum benefit of the doubt. He had a brain that functioned well. Sometimes you get hung up with kids who won't make it. But in his case, it was never clear he wasn't going to."

"He deceived us. We thought he would be our miracle baby," said Amy. "Phil Sunshine says, 'You go into this work with both a heart and a mind.' We all got to the point where we were looking at Matthew with our hearts and not our minds."

When Amy walked out of the hospital at about ten that night, she looked up at the stars and thought, Matthew is finally resting.

Four days later, a memorial service was held in the hospital chapel. The Cordells wanted it there because, as they pointed out, aside from them, his son had only had his Stanford family. A pack of uncles, cousins, and others—most of whom had never visited—crowded in, along with the three primary and some of the other nurses, a parent who had become a friend of the Cordells, Kathy Petersen, and the patient representative who had helped Matthew work out his insurance problems. She had a baby son who was born just a day before Matthew Jr. and who was now a healthy twenty-three pounds—almost five times heavier than Matthew ever got to be.

The unfamiliar relatives all wore black and stood on one side of the chapel. The parents wore bright colors—Sophie in yellow,

Matthew in a suit with a pink shirt and a maroon tie. They explained they wanted to acknowledge the life Matthew had had.

Several people spoke. A minister said a prayer. The parents spoke of their gratitude for the everyone's efforts on their child's behalf. It was not just their son's suffering that had ended, it was also their own. The sorrow they felt was alleviated by the relief of at last having a conclusion. "Matthew kept them together," observed one of the ICN staff, "but he was also a cloud that hung over their lives."

Nursery staff who had come to care for Matthew also felt sorrow mixed with relief. Kathy came away from the service with her grief unspent. "There is so much tragedy in this unit and you never stop," she said. "You fill the bed and go on. I wanted to go and be sad. It was a good service, I guess, though I'll have to be sad on my own."

The medical center disposed of the baby's remains.

It was hard for Amy to come to work the next day and to take on a new baby, another preemie. She wanted to talk about Matthew, but for other nurses on that shift it was just another working day. Some asked her if she would assume primary nurse responsibilities for another infant, committing herself to special attention to a new baby. She declined. How could she have accepted? She would not be ready for that kind of involvement for a long time; she would just have to take day-to-day assignments for a while.

Less than a month after Matthew's death, one of the staff remarked, "He came so close to going home. But when he died, it all fell into place. I guess you know, the parents are splitting and she's going back to Texas."

Did Matthew Cordell really decide to live, and then to die? Did he set the timing? Did he really choose? Or is that idea just the necessary fantasy that permits those who work in the intensive care nursery to continue?

Were his life and suffering futile? Was the expenditure of $530,409.66 on his care justified? Keeping this baby alive for one day cost as much as it would have cost to provide free visits to well-baby clinics for eighty to one hundred children. How many could have been immunized for that sum?

Such questions are important to consider, but they are not for those in the nursery to resolve. In the ICN, the choices exist within the parameters of the resources that have been made available. Reflections on the broader picture seem abstract, whereas Matthew Jr., Sophie, and Matthew Cordell Sr. are real.

The history of Matthew Cordell demonstrates several aspects of the dilemma presented by infants on the threshold of viability. For one, it shows how difficult it is to draw the line between helping and injuring such infants. The physicians never confronted a clear, unambiguous choice with this baby. Were the surgeons too cautious in waiting for improvement in his respiratory status before attempting to repair his hernias? Were they right in believing that morphine was a factor in preventing that improvement from occurring? Did the improvement after hernia repair prove that Matthew might have done better if the surgery had come earlier? Nobody can say for sure. Too little is known about such tiny premature infants. As Dr. Ariagno observed in connection with Angela Walker-Shaw, one of the realities of the ICN is that physicians must always work in an aura of uncertainty.

The public debate about decisions on life's threshold often assumes that physicians know the consequences of alternative courses of action. It assumes that decisions are made in terms of whether infants are deemed "worth saving." In fact, in the case of this baby—as with most others whose hold on survival is extremely tenuous—there was no life-or-death decision. The outcome evolved from a series of medical choices made in light of such facts and experience as were available to physicians and of the baby's perceived best interest. Many of these choices could have tipped the delicate balance between life and death. At the end, the only choice was whether to prolong Matthew's dying or to let him go.

How the problem of uncertainty is weighed depends on many factors, including the individual physician's philosophy and degree of experience, the role of parents, the prevailing moral, economic, and legal climate, the accessibility of resources, and the degree of involvement with a baby.

At birth, a 50 percent chance of survival is considered enough to obtain transfer of an infant from a community hospital to an intensive care nursery and to begin aggressive treatment. Sometimes, a chance of 25 percent or less is considered to be sufficient to justify heroic measures at birth. The odds are affected by many factors, including the place of birth. If a hospital in Reno, say, should call and ask if Stanford would accept a twenty-five-week fetus/baby about to be delivered there to a mother infected with herpes, the answer might be negative, because the transfer would almost surely be fatal to the baby. Were such a baby born in the hospital, however, efforts would be made in its behalf until they were judged clearly futile, though its survival chances would be less than 25 percent.

The degree of certainty demanded for withholding or withdrawal of aggressive treatment increases with the length of time a child has been in the nursery and the degree of personal experience with caregivers. After a time, the slightest glimmer of hope is sufficient to justify continuation of aggressive measures.

Statistically, Matthew's chances of survival at birth were perhaps 25 percent, about the same as the Walker-Shaw twins'. Those chances dimmed with the severity of his illness. But after he had lived for a few months, his caregivers were "enmeshed," as some of the doctors put it. They had invested themselves in the baby to such a degree that they would have required almost 100 percent certainty to stop trying.

Dr. William Benitz, the fourth rotating attending neonatologist at Stanford, calls the phenomenon "the fist in the tar baby": once involved, one is driven to try harder. In the Brer Rabbit story, the tar baby is placed in the rabbit's path to teach him a lesson about his arrogance. In neonatology, Dr. Benitz says, "Unfortunately, it is often the parents' fist that we put in the tar baby."

But medical treatment is only one of several factors that may explain why some borderline babies live and thrive, as Angela did, while others, including Matthew, die. The unique endowment of each baby and the social conditions of home and hospital must be considered.

The role of the infants themselves in the outcome can only be speculated on. Each human being seems to arrive with her or his own particular quantum of life energy. Each is also affected by the degree and quality of the care she or he receives. Some babies simply don't grow, though no organic explanation is found. Researchers have identified the syndrome among both human and simian infants, linked it with maternal neglect, and called it nonorganic failure to thrive. Other babies, despite heavy odds against them, do well if there is a strong positive interaction with parents.

It would be exacerbating injustice to suggest that Matthew's parents were at fault. But they visited him far less frequently than the Shaws visited their baby. Nor did the Cordells—being less familiar with hospital procedures and staff—hound caregivers daily. Despite everyone's best intentions, the old saw that the squeaky wheel gets the grease may have had some relevance in this setting as well.

Angela's parents lived nearby; Matthew's were many miles away. Angela's set their own schedules; Matthew's had jobs with rigid time boundaries. Angela's family was stable and comfortable; Matthew's was going through wrenching transitions, emotionally and financially stressed. Angela's mother had excellent prenatal care, rest, and family support during her pregnancy; Matthew's mother's prenatal care clearly left much to be desired. Matthew's parents both worked long hours, went to weekend classes, and cared for two other children without extended family help. It is not impossible—though, of course, it cannot be proved—that Matthew might have been born at term if he had had the advantages of Angela's home and medical environment.

Was it fair to Matthew and his family to try so hard to keep him alive? Sophie was one of the many mothers whose temperament may not lend itself to the enormously difficult task of nurturing a marginal infant. She already felt guilt-ridden because of the baby's prematurity, as many mothers, irrationally, do. If the child had died at home, that burden of guilt would have grown. What would have been the effect on her other children? Matthew's survival would have added to the family's financial instability, leading to Sophie's having to give up her job and consequently the possible loss of the house. The alternative would have been to send Matthew to foster care.

From the point of view of the infant, his family, and society, was it fair to spend half a million dollars the way it was spent on Matthew Cordell? His caregivers can only reply that he had a chance. The question is for others to answer. Matthew's account, however, must be placed beside that of miracle infants like Angela Walker-Shaw when policymakers choose how to allocate public resources.

CHAPTER SIX

The Price of

Misunderstanding

Among some of the Spanish-speaking farm and factory workers in the great agricultural valley south of Palo Alto, the Stanford Medical Center has a reputation for being a place where doctors use ignorant people's children for experiments. Social workers and physicians have heard that rumor now and then from parents. But none of the doctors who became involved with Maria de Jesús Rodriguez realized that her mother and grandmother believed it. Had they known, the tragedy might have been averted.

The most terrible fact about Maria's plight—and that of her fragile young family—however, is that it was foreseen. People in the hospital knew what was coming in advance. Yet nobody stopped the progress of the disaster, Maria was forced to live when she was clearly trying to die. Why? By whose will and directive?

No simple answer can be offered. What happened was shaped by what the people involved with the baby understood, by what they knew from their own experience and failed to know about each other. All the participants were of good will. All tried to do what was best for the baby. But, as in the ancient Indian tale about five blind men and an elephant, each perceived only a part of a larger pattern and generalized from that about the whole. At the heart of this tragedy was what may be called a communications gap—a euphemism for a failure of compassion. The opposite of compassion is cruelty. Yet everyone cared and nobody can really be blamed.

. In the hospital records, Maria's history begins in July 1984, with the transport of her nineteen-year-old mother, Camilla, from a town in the the San Joaquin Valley while she was in labor. Three weeks earlier, her placenta had become detached and her membranes had ruptured prematurely. When she arrived in the delivery room, no fetal heart tones could be detected. A Caesarean section was performed. At delivery Maria weighed 950 grams, about two pounds two ounces, and was judged to be of about twenty-seven to twenty-eight weeks' gestational age. She had been severely asphyxiated, showed respiratory distress, and had seizures. By the standard physical assessment at birth, the Apgar score, she was in serious trouble. Cardiopulmonary resuscitation was administered.

The baby did poorly in the nursery. After two weeks, it was clear that she had a malformed kidney, an abnormal heart valve, and other problems. Three EEGs indicated that damage to the nervous system was so extreme that the child's chance of any kind of autonomous life was minimal. At best, she might be trainable.

The attending physician called a meeting of the ethics committee. Those present included physicians from the intensive care nursery and obstetrics, nurses, and a social worker. Their consensus that intensive care be withdrawn was presented to the family. The parents refused to accept the hopelessness of the situation and asked that everything possible be done to keep the baby alive.

Subsequently, the attending neonatologist asked for another meeting, for he was of the opinion that further intensive care was medically contraindicated and was concerned that the family might not have understood. The father, Richard Rodriguez, the mother, Camilla, and the maternal grandmother came. The physician was careful to make clear that he had no doubts about the bleak outlook for the baby. Richard seemed to accept the situation but felt his wife should decide. The grandmother insisted that more could be done. The physician perceived the grandmother and mother as defiant and felt they were putting their own needs before the baby's.

The physician tried to make the case to the family from Maria's point of view, pleading for mercy in her behalf. He told them that he, too, was a Catholic, and would be interested in having the Catholic chaplain talk to them if they were confused by what he was explaining. They did not take up the offer but continued to insist that everything possible be done. The physician felt that the grandmother was the one who was making the decision and that she had erected a wall of unreason against the information he was doing his best to impart. Finding no way to penetrate it, he finally felt compelled to give up. Later, reflecting on that meeting, he thought that his only other option would have been to go to court, arguing in the baby's behalf on the ground of wrongful life.

The concept of wrongful life had been advanced in court for infants who were kept alive by technological means although it was unrealistic to expect that they would ever outgrow their extreme disabilities. No court had thus far explicitly acknowledged the validity of this concept, but further consideration was almost assured.[1] The doctor knew that someday he might have to take a stand on the issue, in behalf of a newborn patient. But, for numerous reasons, this case was not appropriate for such a battle.

Others in the nursery were as distressed as the senior physician by the continuing heroic treatment of this extremely damaged infant, but saw the Rodriguezes as confused and mistrustful rather than defiant. "The parents are really simple people," said a fellow. "They seemed to have the idea that the doctors wanted to kill the baby because they did not want her. They wanted us to keep her until we could make her well. And if we couldn't, they said they still wanted us to continue supporting her but did not want her to suffer too much. So we're supporting her."

"How do you feel about that?" he was asked.

"I don't feel right," he said. "I don't feel we're doing anything for society, for the family, or for the baby. I've made vegetables before."

Treatment was escalated. Among other things, digitalis was given to stimulate the heart. Various other pharmacological measures were taken. When, at rounds, a new intern looked askance, someone explained that the parents wanted everything possible done.

The nurses had no hope for Maria. They found it difficult and depressing to take care of her, to jam the tubes down her throat, poke her, and suction her when her future looked so bleak. "Intensive care works, but it's not for every baby," said one nurse. "I can't do much for her. It's very frustrating. She's been screaming for two hours." Though the endotracheal tube (ET) running between the vocal cords prevented Maria from making a sound, the nurse heard her silent scream in the violent contortions of her body and mouth and the rapid jiggles on the monitor screen, indicating a rapid heart beat. "She seems to have become immune to the tranquilizer she's been on," the nurse said as she removed the ventilator tubes to suction the baby in an effort to give her some relief. Then, with another nurse holding Maria's head, she bagged her and once again hooked her up to the breathing machine. "Look, she already has cerebral palsy." The baby's legs were trembling in what one of the doctors on rounds had termed miniature CP. The nurse bundled Maria tightly into her blanket. "And now they're talking about heart surgery," she said. "I think the parents don't understand."

The parents rarely came. Had they managed to visit more frequently, perhaps the misunderstanding would have been discovered in time and events might have taken a different course. But they remained strangers to most of the staff involved with their baby, though they kept in close touch with the nurses by telephone. So nobody in the ICN understood why the mother and grandmother had fiercely refused to hear what the doctors tried to tell them at the beginning of Maria's life. Nor did the parents learn to trust the ICN doctors.

When Maria was two and a half months old, physicians sought to move her to the hospital closest to her family's home. But that hospital had only a Level II nursery and it would not accept her unless she managed to free herself of the respirator. A senior physician then proposed surgery to repair the damaged arterial valve that was impeding blood flow, in hopes that, if the infant survived, her breathing would improve. Without such surgery, there was a strong possibility that she would die of chronic lung disease or its complications.

The proposed surgery was discussed among the doctors. All three attendings had by now been involved with Maria. The doctor who had been especially distressed by her family's attitude was ambivalent. Even if this operation was successful, it would do nothing to alleviate the baby's profound neurological and other deficits. But he recognized that, given the parents' expressed wish for maximum treatment, something had to be done to get Maria off the ventilator. He therefore agreed to the surgery, stipulating that the parents be at the hospital when it took place. Another parents' conference was scheduled, to explain the plan and obtain parental consent.

Maria's daytime primary nurse, Vanessa, was astonished when she heard that surgery was being considered. It made no sense at all to her, given the baby's condition. She thought the plan was the brainchild of some surgeon from outside the ICN, and that the neonatologists would be against it. On the morning of this conference, Vanessa was quite certain of what would transpire: "I don't think the parents will have any choice" she stated. "Camilla's a teenaged mother who already has two other kids. It will be presented to the parents that a heart operation is not what is best for the baby." Vanessa, who had been taking care of Maria since her birth, had come to know and like the parents, mostly over the telephone.

The Rodriguezes arrived. Camilla, a diminutive girl, looked like a typical high school student. Her light brown hair, which had been blow-dried to an attractive curl, framed a pretty, intelligent face with light blue eyes. She wore a striped T-shirt with a white collar, jeans, and tennis shoes. Richard, somber in aspect and very pale, wore a black suit. He stood very straight and his severe silence suggested that he was attempting to cover up his total bewilderment.

Camilla bent over the incubator with a glowing smile, as though looking at a wonderful birthday present rather than at the tragic little daughter the transparent box contained. This was incongruous unless one knew that Camilla's mother had advised her that, if she wanted the baby to get well, she must be sure to send only good feelings toward her. Along with fearful fantasies about the hospital, the mother had imparted to Camilla the idea that faith, positive feelings, and loving care could effect the child's cure.

The nurse reached into the incubator to pick up Maria and hand her to Camilla to hold. She talked to Camilla. When the attending physician appeared, Vanessa accompanied him and the parents into the parent conference room. Before long, all three were back. Vanessa, visibly upset, was talking earnestly with the young couple. Camilla was upset. Richard looked blank. The operation would be performed. That day, at her own request, Vanessa went off Maria's case. Being professionally correct, she was careful to keep this information from the parents.

What was happening troubled the nurse greatly. "Every system of this baby is damaged. She is severely brain damaged," she said. "The parents know. I made sure they know that this baby is probably not going to see and hear, is not going to walk. I've talked with them. They don't want extraordinary measures. They say, 'We'll take her home and take care of her.' What else are they going to say? They want what's best for the baby."

Vanessa said that originally the parents wanted everything done. They did not believe the doctors' assessment of their baby. But since then, as the baby failed to sustain breathing without a ventilator, and as they saw that she was in pain, they had begun to wonder whether she really could recover and whether they were being selfish in wanting her to live. Vanessa felt that the case for the proposed surgery was presented in a way that left the parents only the option of consent.

The nurse was convinced that the parents were ready to do whatever the doctors recommended. They would be willing to let her go. "But if the attending physician says, 'We think she deserves every chance,'" she said emotionally, "how can you possibly say no?

"Of course," she added, "the doctors are human, too, and they want to believe that what they do is best for the child. But neonatology has really changed these past five years. In the new emphasis on 'what's best for the child,' you're not allowed to consider the effect on the rest of the family. And best for the child is taken to mean that whatever shred of life there is, now, is better than no life because death is irreversible."

Though she was aware that, in the Rodriguez case, the bioethics committee had earlier found that discontinuance of aggressive treatment was a reasonable option, she felt that the proposed heart surgery was indicative of a tendency to lean too much toward intervention.

"Eleven years ago, when I started working in the ICN, the attitude was very different. When it was obvious that an infant would suffer severe brain damage that we felt, through our tests, was irreversible and extreme, there was a lot of attention to what the parents felt. An infant would not be kept alive mechanically against the parents' wishes. But now, with the new [federal] regulations, the input from parents is given very little weight in similar cases," she said, "while any indication from parents that they want full support is given a great deal of weight." She was suggesting that it was easier to misinterpret confusion and ambivalence and to misread it as a wish that everything be done. For the doers, that course was safer.

Vanessa said she had withdrawn from the case because she could not in good conscience participate in unnecessary suffering. Other nurses interpreted Vanessa's withdrawal as burnout. One of the neonatologists believed she had misunderstood the physicians' predicament. But however others interpreted her action, the fact was that Vanessa's view of the baby's best interests, and her description of those interests to the parents, was radically different from the view of the attending neonatologist who had met with the parents that day.

To this doctor, the earlier ethics committee meeting was now history. He viewed Maria as a ventilator-dependent infant who needed to get off the breathing machine, whose future was discouraging but not certain. "The child may be viewed as a child with certain disabilities," he said. "Whether these disabilities will become handicaps or not depends on how society can meet the needs of that individual . . . She could have some degree of spasticity, the extent of which would not be certain. It might be a disability. How handicapping it would be is unclear. The prognosis for her intellectual development is entirely a matter of speculation. So what you have is someone who has suffered a series of events, who may show, on the physical examination, evidence of some neuromuscular problem. But the severity of that is unclear. Nobody can tell you how severe it is at this point.

"The baby has an abnormal EEG, but plenty of people with abnormal EEGs are normal individuals, so the EEG by itself is not a clear prognosticator. It may indicate that a certain proportion of babies tested will have a bad prognosis but that means that another proportion will not. Even with all that information, a certain amount of uncertainty is left, which is why people continue to try to help the individual—because you don't know whether at the very mildest the person may need to wear glasses and have a leg brace and that's it."

Arguing by exception rather than probability, the physician had arrived at a conclusion that obliged him to press on. But what did the burden of facts suggest? he was asked. "The burden of facts suggests that she may be not only disabled but that she will have significant handicaps that will not be remediable." The operation would not change that situation.

He had told the parents that some injury had occurred to Maria's brain, he said, but that he could not tell whether she would recover from it and where along the spectrum of possible disabilities she might arrive.

His commitment was to the dim ray of hope, the small quotient of uncertainty that nearly always remains, even when the burden of evidence predicting a terrible outcome seems, to others, overwhelming. From a certain perspective, this is a heroic attitude. It's the attitude we have been taught to admire: the hero never gives up; the hero is undaunted by the odds. But in this situation, might not such a commitment, if narrowly focused, have obscured the wider picture of the child in the family setting? If the alternatives were recovery or death, there would be no moral problem. But what if the ray of hope was a mirage and the infant survived, as seemed likely, in a state that was, in effect, between life and death? What of her and her family then?

The reason for Camilla's sickly look soon became apparent. Added to the troubles with the baby was a new and more familiar concern: the family would be evicted if money was not soon found to pay the rent. Like many of their neighbors, the Rodriguezes depended on seasonal work in the food-processing industry. It was autumn and the canneries had begun to lay people off. Richard, with three years' seniority, was kept on longer than many others, but his paycheck had been cut in half. Soon he, too, would be laid off for the season. Camilla was sick with worry. She had lost weight, her face was drawn, her hair no longer had its bounce and sheen.

"The rent on this place is $350 a month," she said, sitting in her living room one morning soon after the hospital visit to discuss heart surgery for Maria. "When Richard first started working, he got $9.98 an hour. But last week he went down to another bracket, at $5 an hour. He works ten P.M. to six A.M., five days a week, as before, but he brings home only $178 a week, instead of $350. It's not enough. I have five days until I have to pay the rent. He has $178 coming Friday, but that will only be half, and it leaves nothing for living. I have $150 in layaway for the baby and I can't take that out. As it is, I'm already running low on food. All last week we ate beans and rice, potatoes and beans."

She lit a cigarette and gulped the smoke. Her hand showed a faint tremor. "Besides rent, there's the light bill, $35. It's high because everything in this house is electric. Then there's $13 a month at the Laundromat. With $178, we have to save three of his checks for rent and of the last, half goes to bills and we have not much left for groceries. I'm scared."

The day Richard's pay was cut, Camilla went to apply for welfare. To reduce the waiting period from forty-five days to thirty, she told the social worker her husband had left. "I'll have him not-in-the-home until I get the money, then I'll report him back in the home. He'll go stay with his dad," she explained. With the baby, she would get $700 a month. If she found a part-time job, welfare would drop to $350, but she might still be ahead. She had put in applications at stores and restaurants in the vicinity and hoped to be hired by one of them in three or four weeks, when the Christmas season began.

But right now the question was how to get through the month, how to hold on to the house so they would not all have to move in with Richard's father again. She couldn't bear it, especially now, with Maria. "Jumping from house to house, that's how it was for me," she said. "I don't want that for my kids. I'm trying to give them a better life."

Four-year-old Dicky and three-year-old Tamina were wrestling on the living room floor. The TV was flashing cartoons, but neither the children nor Camilla seemed to notice. She rose from the couch to shoo them out of the house.

Though spare, the house was tidy. Above the television set, which was the focal point of the room, hung a blue velvet painting of a girl with hair blowing across her face, a tear rolling down her left cheek, and a unicorn behind her. Below, under the videocassette player, was a shelf with votive candles, a glass filled with coins and a few dollar bills, and a picture of Maria in a crocheted frame.

"So all I can do now is wait," said Camilla, returning. "For the welfare, for a job, for the baby. And the longer I wait the more scared I get. At night, I can't sleep. When Richard comes home after six in the morning, I'm barely falling asleep. I'm always nervous, thinking, How about if the light man comes to turn off the light? How am I going to feed my kids and give them a bath? And the baby, how about the baby?"

Her mother used to lie awake, listening for her husband's return, wondering whether this would be one of the nights when he would drag her out of bed in a drunken rage while the children clung together, holding hands, in the next room.

"Since the money's dropped, we've been arguing," Camilla continued. "Like Richard says, knowing Maria will come home and we don't have money, it's hard. I got Pampers and a crib but I can't get the layaway. And we're always arguing about going to see her. I want to go but our car isn't running. Even if it did, it would cost for gas. There's a free bus that goes twice a week to all the hospitals near San Francisco. It leaves at seven A.M., stops in Oakland, San Francisco, and gets to Stanford about noon. Then it leaves at one P.M.. So you travel all day and get to stay an hour. And meanwhile Richard or someone has to take care of the kids."

Richard has a "short fuse," she said, so she tries to deal with things that upset him, like bills. When things go wrong, he gets mad at her. But he has learned, she said, to go out and take a walk to calm down instead of blowing up at her. She has warned him that she would not be like her mother, who put up with her father's beatings for nineteen years, until he threw her out of a moving van one night, shattering her arm and finally prompting her to take the four children and leave him. Richard was not like that. He did not have a drinking problem.

Camilla had been in the ninth grade when her mother left her father. She had been doing fine, especially in science and math, even though they moved around so much that she never stayed in any school for a full term. But after they left her father, she began to act out. She cut school, stayed out late, got drunk. Eventually she was picked up by the police and sent to juvenile hall.

"And then my mom did something I could not forgive her for," said Camilla. "She asked the counselors, before they let me go, to cut my hair. See, I had my hair long, real long, past my knees. My mom knew how I cared for my hair. I used to get up early just to mess with it. And they cut it real short and blunt. I said, 'At least braid it and let me have my braid,' but they said no."

Her mother may have wanted to save Camilla from the path her older sister had already taken: pregnancy followed by marriage. But if so, the haircut either did not help or had the opposite effect. "I admired my sister because she did not have to put up with my mom no more. But then, when I got pregnant I realized I had lost one boss and gained two. I now had to put up with the baby and his dad." Camilla smiled.

Richard had grown up with Hispanic gangs in Los Angeles and San Jose. He was in the eleventh grade, doing well enough to expect to graduate, but when he learned he was about to become a father he dropped out. He disappeared for four months, then returned. They married.

After the second child, Tamina, was born, Camilla decided to be fitted with an intrauterine birth control device. She thought she might be able to go back to school to learn to be a bookkeeper or have some other "desk job." But the device caused an infection and had to be removed. Soon after, she was again pregnant, with Maria.

145

"I thank God Richard stuck with me," Camilla said. "He could have left me; most guys that age do. But he stayed with me, with Dicky, and when Tamina was born he still stayed with me, and now the baby is here and he's sticking with me still."

It was a long way from the world Camilla and Richard inhabited to the multimillion-dollar research hospital in Palo Alto where their baby languished. They were separated by geography, but even more by education, economics, and culture. What the young couple had heard about big medical centers from people they knew, or what they had gleaned and surmised from various sources, led them to believe that marvels could be accomplished there, but that nefarious practices went on as well. Or rather, it was Camilla who had this suspicion. Richard, basically, went along.

What Camilla thought she heard the doctors say was as remote from what they actually said as her life was from the doctors'. "They wanted us to sign her over to the state so they could take her to a mental hospital and experiment on her until she died," Camilla said, sitting up straight. "But Richard and I said, 'No way.' No way they would hurt her more than she is hurting already. We said, 'You do what you can for her and we'll take her home and take care of her. We'll take her as she comes.'"

There was no problem here with language. Maria's parents were both natives of the United States. But the misunderstanding could not have been more profound. Camilla got the impression that since her baby was so damaged, and since she and Richard were poor, from the Valley, and did not fully understand what was going on, the doctors did not consider it worth their while to try to make Maria well; that they wanted the parents' consent to let their baby be used for experiments, like a laboratory animal. Camilla was horrified and said no, thereby setting into motion a seemingly inexorable process that would keep this baby on the threshold of death for many months, leading her to live out the doctors' grim prognosis. (Later, when she heard that a baboon heart had been transplanted into a newborn infant named Fae, Camilla would say, "They're using her as a guinea pig—just like they wanted to do with Maria. Those doctors should be sent to jail!")

Camilla's notion that hospitals use human babies as laboratory animals seemed to have grown from what she had heard from her mother about her younger sister, who had also been small and premature and who had grown up to be an A student in college. According to Camilla, "They had all kinds of doctors trying to convince my mother to sign my sister over to the state so they could take her to a mental institution." Within the strangeness of the entire medical center environment, that notion seemed credible to her.

The first meeting with the doctors was overwhelming for both Camilla and Richard. The way she remembered it, "We went to the conference room and there were six doctors following right behind, and six nurses." There were actually only a few people present. "We went there thinking there was nothing wrong. And then they were saying Maria had all these problems. And I started crying. I said, 'Wait a minute. Back up. When I was calling every day the nurses said she was fine. Now you tell me this?'"

What the nurses actually had told Camilla cannot be verified. But the likelihood is that they were cautious and nonspecific. Parents of newborn sick babies—even professional people—commonly fail to accept news about their children's condition on the first round.

Unprepared for the doctors' deathly prognosis, Camilla concluded there was foul play afoot. In the turmoil of information and emotion, in this alien place, faced with alien authorities, she reached for her mother's warnings and heard in the doctors' explanations: "'We can keep her alive if you want us to, or you can sign papers giving her over to the state.' So I figured, they don't want to waste their time on her when they can just sign her over to the state and take her to a mental institution so they can be experimenting on her. So I freaked out and I said, 'No. I'll just keep her, if she's slow or whatever.' And the doctors said, 'Okay, but we told you straight out.'"

In fact, nobody asked the parents to sign the baby over to the state. The doctors had tried to make clear that, for this child, aggressive treatment might do more harm than good. They had asked the parents whether, under the circumstances, they consented to the doctors not doing all they knew how to do. Would Camilla have acted differently if she had understood?

147

"I would have understood if they had said it that way to me, but they didn't," Camilla replied. "I would have said, 'Fine. If it's going to do her more harm than help her, then just go ahead and let her die, if it's not going to help her.' I would have said that."

But because Camilla failed to grasp the meaning of what she was told, because the doctors' words fell into a perceptual milieu that warped their meaning, Maria's fate was set on the slippery slope. From then on she would be the subject of continuing and increasing interventions that would keep her in a perilous and painful predicament for a long time to come. Consequently, Camilla's frail young shoulders would take on an additional burden so big that it would stretch her strength beyond its limits.

"After that conference, I was crying and crying. Camilla, what are you going to do? What are you going to do? I went out and called my mom. She said, 'Camilla, don't sign no papers. And the most important thing, when you see the baby, don't cry, don't feel hurt. Don't feel sorry for her. The more you cry and feel sorry for her, the more she feels it and she'll just give up. When you're there, talk to her and give her hope so she can keep fighting.'"

"And I haven't. Up to this day I pray to God. My mom told me to 'cut the tail off the baby,' to baptize her. We did. And then we went to church and lit a bunch of candles."

Nobody at the hospital knew why the parents had asked that "everything be done." One of the doctors continued to think of their demand as defiant. Nurses, who sensed there was a different explanation, never dreamed what had been in this mother's mind.

In the nursery, where the intensity of the present obscures the larger view, Maria's early history was of academic interest by the time the heart surgery took place. She was viewed as a ventilator-dependent baby and the issue was how to get her off. The operation proved to be a success. Maria extubated herself shortly thereafter and continued breathing without machine support.

Later, a social worker who was close to the case said that she had never heard anyone explain the neurological situation to the parents in detail. The social worker had heard doctors telling the Rodriguezes that the baby would have serious problems, that she would not have the same life as other children, that she might need special schooling. But it was all said in a general way, leaving much room for distortion. To that, one of the neonatologists replied that the social workers usually make sure that the physicians' explanations are comprehensible to families.

The nurses had tried to explain the baby's condition to Camilla and Richard by pointing out symptoms of neurological damage: the twitching of the baby's feet, for example. "But," the social worker said, "when you are very young, come from such a different background, and have a choice between people at this hospital and your own mother, who says, 'Just talk with her, don't give up and she will be like your sister who is an A student in college,' isn't it to be expected you would listen to your mother? This is going to be one of our disasters, believe me. You feel rage. And there is nobody to blame. It's the system."

The vision of her successful sister, which Camilla's mother had placed before her, was not realistic. Maria could not be like her. Nor could Camilla carry out her mother's command that she bring only positive feelings toward the baby. She was smoking two and a half packs of cigarettes a day and weighed only eighty-two pounds. Her size-eight jeans hung so loosely they would have fallen off without the belt. Worries buzzed inside her head all the time and she was getting headaches. The tremor in her hands was worse.

She felt responsible for the baby's condition in some vague way, and she felt guilty about not going to see her as often as she should have. She feared that when Maria came home she might do something wrong and cause her to die. She blamed herself for everything else that went wrong: the fights with Richard, the fact that they had no money even though he had worked all he could and had not spent anything on himself. He did not smoke, drink, or go out with friends. His life was at home. He had not abandoned her and the children. Yet Camilla had not been able to keep food in the refrigerator and the bill collector from the door. And now she had to be positive and cheerful for the baby.

The Rodriguezes were what social workers call, in their depersonalized jargon, a multiproblem family. All that held it together was jerry-rigged and likely to tumble any day, for any number of reasons. Camilla's daily life was a continuous struggle to keep the various components together. It is the kind of struggle that people who did not grow up knowing about the culture of poverty seldom understand. It uses up whatever quotient of hope exists and turns all plans and intentions into broken promises. Success is getting through the current crisis, and there is a new crisis daily.

The rent crisis was temporarily resolved—or deferred for a month, anyway—by a tactic many poor families resort to—doubling up. A woman with a ten-year-old daughter moved into the small house and paid part of the rent. But then she refused to chip in for food, kept eating, and was asked to leave.

The car did not run because somebody had stolen the battery and they could not afford another. The welfare check was slow in coming, and neither Camilla nor Richard could find work to make up for the loss of income. Then Richard fell sick. The morning he came home after being laid off for the season, he collapsed on the kitchen floor. Camilla woke as he came in the front door, heard him go to the refrigerator and open a can of Seven-Up. Then she heard the crash as he, having passed out, fell. It was a scene she had often experienced with her father, but with Richard the cause was not alcohol; it was an injured lung that had collapsed.

This had happened before. Camilla dragged her husband to the couch, put wet cloths around his head, and when he came to, went for a neighbor to take him to the doctor. Richard returned with penicillin, pain killer, and sleeping pills. Usually the doctor gave him some oxygen and he improved. His lungs were scarred. One of the doctors he had seen thought they might have been damaged by chemicals, but Richard did not think he had been exposed to anything very toxic, except chlorine when he worked as cleanup man in a cannery. It was lucky, thought Camilla, that this had not happened at work, while he was sitting on top of a ladder, sending fruit down a chute.

In a multiproblem family, appointments are often forgotten in the intensity of the struggle to get through the day. Days can go by unnoticed. Camilla broke appointments at the hospital, creating the impression among the staff that she either did not care about her baby or was irresponsible.

In November, when Maria was five months old, she was judged stable enough to do without the resources of a Level III nursery and transferred to a hospital in the family's hometown.

In the smaller hospital everything seemed older and more worn—the carpet in the lobby, the furniture and equipment, the nurses, the physician who shuffled in wearily and did rounds alone. In the much smaller acute care nursery, no physician was present around the clock; there was only one on call. The sound of pulsing monitors was louder than it had been at Stanford. There were no windows. ("What's the weather like?" a nurse asked a visitor. "In here, you have no idea. Sometimes at the end of a twelve-hour shift I'm so strung out I think I'll go crazy. I come out and feel like I'm in a fishbowl.")

Maria was in a much quieter, also windowless intermediate ward with six other babies, all close to going home. She had graduated from an incubator to a bassinet, and she looked much better than some of her roommates, who seemed wizened with age or had deformities. She had become a little person—pretty, with long dark eyelashes and plenty of curly dark hair. But she had not yet reached the weight of a normal baby at birth. At almost six months she was four pounds fifteen ounces.

Under the watchful eyes of a nurse, Camilla performed the routine she would have to repeat every three hours once her baby was home. She turned her on the side, patted her on the back with a rubber device to drain fluid from her lungs. Then she took a flexible plastic tube, dipped it into saline solution, and pushed it down the baby's throat to free it of mucus. "Do it so that it does not touch the mucous membranes and make them bleed," advised the nurse one particular morning. The baby twisted at the unpleasantness.

Next Camilla suctioned the nostrils. Then she inserted another tube into the mouth as far as the stomach and poured in some potassium chloride. After that, she took the baby out of the bassinet, held her close to her breast, and poured formula into the gavage tube. Camilla held Maria until the baby upchucked a little, then wiped her mouth. The baby's eyes were turned to her, with recognition. Camilla sat with her a while, swaying back and forth. Two other mothers arrived, picked up their sad babies, and sat with them, too, in adjacent chairs, gently rocking. They chatted and exchanged theories on what might have gone wrong, or what they might have done wrong, to create their particular calamity.

By mid-December, when Maria was six months old, things took a turn for the better for the entire Rodriguez family. There was a Christmas tree in front of the living room window, decorated with paper chains Dicky had made in the nursery school he had begun to attend mornings. (Tamina had been admitted, but Richard, fearing the child molestors he had heard about on TV, decided she was too young to go.) Richard had recovered and watched the children while Camilla worked. One of the application forms she had filed in September had paid off as a job in a discount dry goods store nearby. It was only part time, at minimum wage, for the Christmas season, but it put a new buoyancy into her walk, a new confidence into her voice.

"It's the first job I ever had and the first thing I ever did on my own," she said one morning, braiding Tamina's hair. "I'm on the cash register part of the time and in the warehouse part of the time. The first part is easy, because all I really do is press buttons; the machine does the tax and tells you how much to give back. I don't like the warehouse as much, because it's too heavy for me, I'm not strong enough." She still weighed less than a hundred pounds.

The biggest news, however, was that Maria was home. Though regular newborn clothes were still too big on her, she was free of lines and needles, her coloring was a wholesome pink, and her tremors were no longer apparent. She finally weighed over five pounds.

"To me she's just a normal baby except that she does not know how to suck and she's small," said Camilla. "She likes to be on her belly on my lap, her head hanging down, and for me to pat her back. She gets a lot of that stuff in her lungs out that way. She knows what sound is. She doesn't hear, I know that, because she doesn't respond to a loud noise even when it's close. But she feels the suction machine vibrate against her bassinet. She doesn't like it. When I turn it on she puts her hands over her face. She doesn't like the gavage tube, either. She'd like to suck, but she does not know how. But she sees and she loves Dicky."

The baby's inability to swallow meant that the feeding tube continued to be necessary. Her condition was still extremely delicate. Since being discharged from the hospital for the first time in her half-year life, she had already been readmitted for a few days, after aspirating some of her food. She still had to be suctioned every couple of hours. This, plus the job and her duties to the other two children, meant that Camilla was getting little sleep. Had she been one of the fortunate parents who have good health insurance, or an adequate income, she would surely have had a nurse in the home to help out. Nevertheless, she was much more cheerful this day than she had been on previous visits.

"I'm just so glad to have her home," she said. "This baby has had too many things done to her. She's had too many needles;

she has too many bruises. When she was in the hospital here I didn't even want to go see her. I didn't want to see those things in her. At Stanford they've got a lot of equipment, but a lot of doctors are just experimenting. I told her doctor now, I don't want anymore. She's been poked enough."

That same day, at exactly noon, while Camilla was out for an hour, a man from the electric company came and turned off the power in the house for nonpayment of bills. Richard had just turned on the broiler to make some hambugers for the children when he saw the man outside the house. He said he told the man about the baby who required electric suctioning. He even took the suction pump outside to show him. But the man said his orders were just to turn off the electricity.

Fortunately, someone on the scene knew what to do to get the power restored and make sure that word about the incident got to higher-ups in the company. The electric wall clock, which had stopped at 12:00, moved again at 1:07, and a smell of broiling meat came from the oven. The power company spokesman said its employee had been questioned and had reported that nobody had told him about the baby's life-support equipment. He said a youth, who looked to be around twenty, had merely said, "I thought we had till the fifteenth." The bill had not been paid since July and $213 was owing.

A month later, when the bill remained overdue, a man from the electric company knocked on the door and did not go to the meter at all. He gave Camilla a card with the name and number of a minister in a social agency that serves disabled children. She called; he found funds to take care of the bill and also set wheels in motion for placing Maria on permanent disability status, for which she could qualify as soon as she reached her first birthday. She would then go on the rolls for life, if need be, as a recipient of Supplemental Security Income (SSI) and get a gold card that would entitle her to free lifelong Medicare.

Three days after Christmas, Camilla saw that her baby was once again struggling desperately to breathe. She rushed Maria to the local hospital, with what seemed to be viral pneumonia. Maria spent two weeks there. This time, Camilla did not want to visit. "I did not want to see her with all those things in her again," she said. Because Maria lost weight, continued to have trouble breathing, and would not tolerate her feeds, the local physician decided to send her back to Stanford. The idea was to see if her feeding could be improved with a gastrostomy, which would allow liquids to be poured directly into the stomach, bypassing the esophagus, which was irritated from the gavage tube. The gastrostomy can be either a temporary or a permanent solution.

The baby's return to Stanford was the start of a whole new series of misunderstandings. Maria, accompanied by Camilla, went by ambulance. But Camilla also left with the ambulance, right away, without signing the necessary papers. Had she missed this ride back, she would have faced a wait of several hours and a long bus ride, because public transportation between Palo Alto and her home town was sparse and circuitous. In fact, she might not have been able to get home until the next day.

A week later, staff were highly annoyed. "They had to cancel the operation," a social worker said. "It was scheduled for yesterday, but the parents have not come or called. They don't have a phone. I called the message phone and the mother just happened to be there. We arranged that [a physician] would call and set a time, but nobody answered.

"So it was arranged that the public health nurse would go to the home. Maybe she could get the mother to give consent. In light of the hostility Camilla had encountered here," she said, "it might be helpful to have the public health nurse act as intermediary. She has lost confidence in us and she needs someone she sees as unthreatening." The social worker was apparently unaware that the confidence problem went way back.

"The trouble started here," she continued, "with the way nurses interpreted her need—not her desire—to leave with the ambulance. That's when the judging started, and it has culminated in the view that she is an indifferent and irresponsible mother. This place does not serve enough poverty-level people to be acquainted with the realities in their lives."

Later, Camilla presented another side of the story. She said she had called the hospital before coming with the ambulance, told whoever answered that she would have to leave right away, and asked that whatever papers she would have to sign be ready. They were not, she said. She also said that she had kept her telephone appointment and had, in fact, waited for the physician's call for more than an hour, but that the physician had called another number, which had been her message phone at an earlier time. Whatever the facts, Camilla had earlier stated that she did not want Maria to have more "things done to her." It was conceivable that the misunderstanding reflected her ambivalence about the proposed gastrostomy.

154

By the time Maria's parents found their way back to Stanford, two weeks after she had been admitted, Maria was gaining weight. An intern had thought to place a gavage tube through her nostril and leave it there, rather than poking it in through the mouth and down her throat for every feeding. This probably reduced the baby's discomfort, and Maria kept her food down. The parents, who had come prepared for another request for consent to surgery, instead were told that a gastrostomy no longer seemed necessary and they could take their baby home. Discharge procedures took so long, however, that they missed the day's only bus to their town. They wrapped the infant in borrowed blankets, covered her face against the winter chill, and caught the public transit bus to San Jose, where they would spend the night with relatives and catch the next bus home in the morning.

It is worth noting that other ICN graduates, with respiratory problems that were not quite as severe as Maria's, were kept indoors, under private nursing care, for the entire winter.

Maria managed to stay home only a few days this time. By early February she was back in the Stanford pediatrics ward, so critically ill that she was intubated again, paralyzed with Pavulon to prevent her movements from interfering with the ventilator, and fed intravenously. After about a week, the paralyzing drug was stopped and she was put on morphine, alternating with Valium. She lay on her back, with IV needles, secured with surgical tape, stuck into her thighs. Her very pale color, with a greenish tinge, indicated that there was a problem with her liver. Heavy secretions from her lungs required frequent suctioning.

Was this not another moment for pausing to reexamine the situation, for weighing whether such heroic measures were still appropriate for a baby who was continually succumbing to lung disease and whose prospects in every other respect were so bleak? The physician in charge said the baby was too sick for decisions to be made on the appropriate course for her. She would have to get better to be evaluated. At this point, he said, it was impossible to tell how bad her lungs were, whether she had a gag reflex, and whether she would be able to swallow. The catch in that, of course, was that once the baby got over the infection, heroic measures would no longer be relevant and the point of a possible decision would have been passed.

Was this not a case now for an ethics committee? The physician thought not. He said he thought that "the hard decisions have to be reached between the parents and the doctor. When you try to take these very hard decisions and spread them over the shoulders of a bunch of people, it winds up being no one's decision."

Yet, in Maria's case, this principle had not worked in practice. It was based on an assumption of trust in the doctor, and on mutual understanding, which had been notably absent from the very beginning.

Had he heard that some of his patients' parents thought Stanford was a place where babies were taken from their families and used for experiments? the physician was asked. Yes, he said, he had, and it troubled him. "A certain socioeconomic group developed this technology. But we have run into some very rough spots between our system and people who come here for care. I sometimes wonder if we are delivering appropriate care. Is this what the families really want? I don't know.

"In the Rodriguez case I might say too much was done. Retrospectively, you can be a genius about such things. But I know that you reach a point when prospectively you can't be sure. So you wind up pressing ahead. Unfortunately, we can't act on what we think the most likely outlook will be." The constraint, he said, is the standard of care. "Most times we press ahead."

So Maria continued to lie on her back, with the blue and white tubes of the respirator attached to her face, her long-lashed eyes gazing at the ceiling. She was still a pretty child, with a strong resemblance to her father, and she was long and very thin. Often, her nurse said, she was "grotesquely agitated, moving like she is riding a bicycle. No, she is not growing, she is using up her energy being mad at the world." With the respirator and the intravenous feeds and various pharmaceuticals, her respiratory infection cleared up; Maria was extubated but still refused to grow. At nine months, her weight continued to hover around five pounds. A gastrostomy was performed, but it did not help her keep her food down. She kept regurgitating and aspirating some of it. Each time that happened, there was a setback, with weight loss.

Two other children, both with birth defects, shared the room with Maria. To her left, a young Hispanic woman with large brown eyes sometimes leaned sadly over a boy with multiple deformities. To her right was a girl about two, with rich black curls, who had a damaged heart and neurological problems and had been in the hospital since her birth, except for one week in a foster home. She had never been able to do anything but lie there, and she would die within the month.

156

"It's a sad room," said the nurse. "All live-ins."

Maria's parents came in once during the first month, on the bus. "I guess they've detached themselves," the nurse went on. But she knew almost nothing about them.

In March, Camilla and the children checked into a home for battered women. The social worker set wheels in motion to place Maria in foster care when she left the hospital. A middle-aged woman came from Maria's hometown to see the baby and receive instruction in her care. She said two of the five children she was caring for also had gastrostomies.

Camilla called from the shelter. She said she and Richard had been fighting constantly about her wanting to go up to Stanford to see the baby. She said she felt guilty about what had happened to Maria and about the possibility she might have to go to foster care. A good mother would not allow that. The social worker she talked with reassured her by saying, "Would a good mother bring a child like Maria into the kind of situation you now find yourself in?"

A month more passed, with Maria still unable to gain weight. Because the gastrostomy had not changed this fact, doctors put in a tube from Maria's nose to her jejunum, the upper part of the intestine, bypassing the stomach, which they hoped would prevent the reflux of the food. They also began to consider yet another operation, to narrow the passage between the esophagus and the stomach, and thus prevent the food from coming back up.

Was it possible that this child simply did not want to live anymore, that she was trying to die? One of the interns said he saw it that way, then shrugged. He was only beginning his apprenticeship at the hospital.

Maria seemed to be going backward. Because she had failed to maintain body temperature, she was placed in an isolette—a highly unusual step with a baby nearing her first birthday. The IVs were moved to her scalp, where some good veins remained. She was very spastic. Her right hand kept brushing the side of her head until it was put in a bandaged splint that sustained an IV; the left went to her mouth. She could not swallow but she loved to suck; she sucked on her fingers all day long.

This was all Maria could do, and it was the only thing that seemed to give her pleasure. But the habit became a cause of conflict between the doctors and the nurses—a conflict that reflected their differing values. Sometimes Maria's fingers would move to her nose and pull out the feeding tube. To prevent that, the doctors put a splint on her left arm, too. Of course, the doctors did not want to deprive Maria of pleasure; they were thinking of the effectiveness of their treatment and the fact that the tube is hard to put back in. They weighed that as more important than whatever satisfaction the sucking gave the baby.

But when they came around again, they would find that the nurses had freed the baby's fingers. "Those fingers are her life," said one of the nurses. "That is the only thing she has." They had developed a strong affection for this pitiful, pretty girl.

The pediatrics ward, where Maria now lived, was only a few dozen feet from the intensive care nursery where she had spent her first five months. But a new set of rotating physicians was now responsible for her. The ICN staff members who had tried to help her in the beginning were aware of her, but no longer involved. "This baby is a tragedy," said one of the neonatologists. Still, he saw no way that he could have dealt with her case any differently than he had done.

As month after month passed, with the baby not strong enough to get out of the incubator, the pediatrics house staff felt increasingly uncomfortable. Maria's was one of those horror stories in which all the arts and techniques doctors learn for the sake of nurturing life and health seemed to have been perverted.

"It's hard to know when to stop," commented a senior resident. "In pediatrics we almost never stop. We get stuck."

But did it make sense to go for yet more surgery in this instance? Was it necessary to narrow the esophageal passage? Why not leave the child a possible way out?

"What are you going to do? Not feed her?" the resident responded, in an obvious reference to the Baby Doe case. Part of the problem, she went on, is the cultural gap. "If she had been from middle-class parents who were educated and spoke good English, I think she would have been treated very differently." She was not implying that there was discrimination against the poor in the hospital. The situation was more subtle. There were times, she explained, when Maria could have been allowed to expire. Despite the many hazards pediatricians face in making a decision not to press ahead with a very sick and damaged baby, many still take a personal risk, if they have the trust and the understanding of the parents. The ethical dilemmas in medicine, and especially in this aspect of it, almost universally involve a breakdown of trust. The breakdown with Camilla was of catastrophic proportions.

Camilla returned to her husband, who promised to go to a counselor. She called the hospital, saying she would be taking her child home after all.

And then, in this continuing tale of sorrow, there was the following dialogue:

"We're going to fight her, of course," said the social worker.

"On what grounds?" she was asked.

"On the ground that the emotional climate in the home is hazardous to the baby's well-being."

In July 1985, Maria, still in the hospital, passed her first birthday. She had become a favorite among the nurses and they festooned her crib with balloons, ribbons, and greeting cards. There was no card from the family. The plan now was to send her to a foster home. She was still in the hospital as summer again turned to autumn. Hospital staff began to talk of her as a possible "failure to thrive," a medical term for a syndrome usually associated with neglect: although no organic explanation can be found, the child simply refuses to grow.

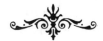

The story of Maria de Jesús Rodriguez raises the question of informed consent. Theoretically, parents are partners in the efforts in behalf of their babies. Their word counts. Ideally, their consent to treatment, or withdrawal of same, is sought and obtained in a manner that allows for understanding and reflection. Ideally, the medical caretakers brief the parents on their child's condition, explain what they propose to do, offer alternatives, and allow them to participate in the decision making.

But there are many barriers between the ideal and its realization. Physicians may explain too much, leaving the parents bewildered under a bombardment of information, or they are too vague, sometimes because they do not know enough and want to be careful, sometimes because they cannot bring themselves to be too blunt, or because they are struggling with an ethical dilemma. Sometimes doctors think they are being clear and simple but do not realize how great the gap is between their expertise and the parents' knowledge of physiology or medicine. Sometimes, under the press of time and other duties, what passes for informed consent is a confused, deferential yes on the telephone or a signature on a line.

For Maria, the physicians tried their best to be clear, as explicit as possible, and to speak to the parents face to face. Because they had to travel so far and found it so difficult to come to the hospital, the parents missed appointments, thereby missing the opportunity to become more knowledgeable about their baby's condition. When they did come, they brought to conferences a perspective that skewed what they were told.

Parents who are grieving for a premature, sick, or damaged child often find it hard to hear physicians' reports, even without prior suspicion about the physicians' intentions. For the Rodriguezes, parental bewilderment was aggravated by their youth, inexperience, and cultural difference. Language was not the problem, but the misunderstanding could not have been greater had they been speaking different tongues. Maria's parents lived in the culture of poverty that is as alien to many Americans as many a distant land.

Camilla's fear that her baby could be used in laboratory experiments was so foreign to the doctors' understanding that no one realized what was in the mother's mind. A basic difference in perception or attitude may not become apparent right away, and there is no common ground for questions. Because the parents and the physicians were so far from communicating with each other, there was no trust. The hospital staff members who thought Camilla was an unreliable and selfish parent did not know what her life was like, or what anguish she experienced because of the baby.

Camilla's is only one tale in which misunderstanding led to tragedy. Many others are known to health professionals. How can they be avoided? The ways are known but they are ignored, not being issues of high priority in hospitals. Informed consent can be reached only with investment of time and attention.

If staff accepted that parents may not understand a difficult message the first time, or even the second, someone should be responsible for continuing the effort at communication until success is reached. Parents' understanding of what they are told can be ascertained by seeking feedback. Simply asking parents to repeat, in their own words, what they have heard could be a positive step.

The physician's presence is often intimidating to parents. It can cause a temporary mental shutdown in people accustomed to venerating a doctor as a powerful authority, so an intermediary could reinforce a message. Camilla had intermediaries: social

workers, sympathetic nurses. They did not know the specific details of Camilla's fears, but they certainly knew that the doctors
were wrong about this young mother's attitude. Physicians remained unaware of the social workers' and nurses' perceptions.

Where geographical and cultural distances are great, an advocate with an awareness of cultural disparities could be helpful.
Recognizing differences, and knowing that they can have profound implications, is the first step toward building an accord.

CHAPTER SEVEN

Death as a

Planned Experience

A Catholic priest who spent eight years serving indigenous villages in Alaska discovered that many of their elderly exerted a remarkable degree of choice over the timing and circumstances of their death. Often when he arrived in response to a summons from a sickbed, he found that preparations had already been made. The dying person had gathered the family and for some days had been praying and telling the story of his life. The house was stocked with food for many people. Soon after taking Communion, the priest later wrote, the person passed on—sometimes within a few hours, sometimes in a matter of days. He particularly remembered one old woman whose death was a community event in which she fully and consciously participated. It was, he found, "a priceless gift to all of us." Reflecting on his experiences, he said, "Dying should be seen as a phase of living and subject to growth, obligations, and opportunities, just as is every other phase of living."[1]

It is widely recognized that people exert a certain amount of control over their dying. Almost everyone knows of wives or husbands who died shortly after their spouse passed on. Often no medical reason is apparent, and those who knew the couple say the cause was a broken heart, or a loss of the will to live. But despite such recognition, our culture—unlike many others—does not, by and large, accept death as a part of life, a spiritual challenge and an opportunity for sharing. There is a tendency to fear, deny, and refuse death, to perceive death as the enemy of life; to shut it out of the mind and, when that is no longer possible, to fight it at all costs.

It is, therefore, ironic yet fitting that the technology we have created for the war against death has forced us to confront it consciously and to choose the time and manner of dying. When does one forgo organ transplants? Kidney dialysis? Heart surgery? When should the respirator be disconnected? In modern medicine, death is often a programmed event.

Since technology can maintain the functioning of a body long after hope of recovery and consciousness have gone, somebody is often obliged to decide when and how death is to occur. Unless that decision is made, the life-support systems become devices that can suspend a person in unlife, much as souls are suspended in Dante's Purgatory.

Karen Ann Quinlan's is the best-known story of such unlife. For ten years after her conscious life ended, she lay in a coma, not clinically brain dead but with no cognitive function. She was kept alive first with a respirator and, when her parents won a court battle to allow her disconnection from the machine, breathing on her own but fed intravenously or through a nasogastric tube. About six months before her death, a judge ruled that the feedings could stop, but her parents could not bring themselves to give such an order. Karen Ann Quinlan died of pneumonia on June 11, 1985, at the age of thirty-one.

The Quinlan decision helped to establish a civil right that the Founding Fathers never thought necessary to secure: the right to die. Since then, several states have passed legislation designed to guarantee this right, mainly by permitting people to write living wills in which they state that they do not want to become objects of heroic life-support measures if they become fatally ill or chronically vegetative, that is, do little more than eat and maintain autonomic functions. (A vegetative patient, unlike a comatose one, has cycles of sleep and wakefulness, opens and closes the eyes, shows facial expressions.)

Although physicians may legally disconnect respirators in hopeless cases, however, our long denial of death has left us without a philosophy to serve as guide for the decisions about time and manner of death that life-extending technologies necessitate. For patients on mechanical life support who do not recover, a moment arrives when the machinery that artificially maintains them becomes useless or begins, irrevocably, to do more harm than good. To recognize that moment is difficult even for the most experienced and gifted physician, but doctors deem it their duty to try. When, consulting with their colleagues, they agree that the moment has arrived, they cease their efforts to save a patient and begin to prepare him and the family for the inevitable. Comfort and the alleviation of suffering become the primary goals.

In the Stanford intensive care nursery, physicians ordinarily prefer to allow infants to die in a parent's arms, free of mechanical attachments. Only if a parent insists, and then only reluctantly, do they keep a baby on the respirator until he actually expires.

Usually, the decision that rescue efforts have failed is made at bedside by the attending physician in consultation with the medical team. But sometimes, when consensus is lacking or when, for some other reason, an attending physician believes that a formal discussion would be useful, the infant bioethics committee is called together.

This committee was organized in 1977 because some physicians, especially Dr. Ronald Ariagno, realized that the required decision making is difficult and confusing, and that ethical issues trouble many physicians, nurses, and others. It became one of the models on which the 1984 federal regulations requiring such committees were based.

At eight o'clock one early spring morning in 1984, the Stanford infant bioethics committee held a meeting to discuss a three-month-old boy, Joshua Patrick, who was the cause of growing anguish for his family and his caregivers. A term baby, he seemed normal except for chest-wall deformities and lungs that were too tiny at birth and did not grow as the rest of his body had grown.

Although his problem was apparent from birth, he was intubated in the delivery room so the best possible diagnosis could be made. The birth defect specialist could not find a specific label for his condition; but no way was found to correct it.

His problem worsened as he grew. He began to suffer extreme air hunger. Several times a day he became frantic, turned dusky, then blue. "His eyes turn up," said one of his nurses. "The look is of someone completely terrified." Nothing could be done to help him until he calmed, which happened as he passed out. At that point, he was revived with oxygen and more ventilation. The more Josh grew and became a person, the harder it was for his nurses to watch him go through this agony, which, in effect, was repeated, daily dying. No hope of recovery was in sight. Yet doctors delayed in taking the irrevocable step.

The situation would have been hard enough with one of the fetus/babies, who are not obviously responsive. But Josh was a full-term three-month-old. "You could talk to him and he would look at you," said his nurse. "As soon as you touched him around the mouth he would cry. He knew you were going to suction him. When you are an adult and they suction you, it feels like they are whisking all the air out of you." He recognized people, smiled at his parents and at others he liked, turned away from others. He batted at toys. "Normally I try not to involve myself too much," said the nurse, "but in this case . . ."

For the family, Josh's survival thus far seemed a miracle, and the longer the boy lived, the more their attachment to him grew. He was his parents' first child; each had another child by a previous marriage. They watched him day by day, and the stress was ripping apart their marriage.

Ethicist Albert Jonson has observed, "We're very good now at producing effects. You put a patient on a respirator, and the effect is that the blood is oxygenated. The effect is almost automatic. The question is, is that effect a *benefit* to the patient? A benefit has to be perceived; it's an appreciated effect."[2]

In the case of Joshua Patrick, the question was becoming increasingly urgent: What was the benefit in continuing life support? Finally, the attending physician, who had held out the longest, waiting for some glimmer of possibility, called the ethics committee meeting. More than a dozen people gathered around a long oak table in the pediatrics department library. They included two of the attending physicians, Dr. Ariagno and Dr. David Stevenson (Dr. Sunshine was on sabbatical), a pediatrics resident on service in the ICN, and a member of the pediatrics faculty who was not part of the ICN, two of the three primary nurses, discharge coordinator Kathy Petersen, a chaplain's representative, a hospital administrator, and a social worker with long experience in the ICN who now worked with disabled children and their families. The committee's composition reflected recommendations of the American Academy of Pediatrics and was in keeping with federal guidelines. Still to be added was a lay person from the community.

Dr. Ariagno made the presentation. The baby had major chest-wall abnormalities and lacked some ribs on his left side. There were muscular and skeletal problems, but the main problem was the lungs, which had shown no growth. The infant had not been able to breathe without extensive mechanical support from the beginning. The question was, Could the lungs enlarge?

Dr. Stevenson said he had searched the literature and found that the baby's problem was "commonly lethal." In most recorded cases, the babies had died in infancy. There were some survivors, but they apparently had a less severe variant of the condition, because it was not recognized until later. "Our approach has been to look at this person as an individual and evaluate his capacities," Dr. Stevenson said.

"What about the parents?" someone asked.

"At the start, the father said, 'If he has no lungs, what are you doing to him?' They felt if we could do something, we should," said the baby's day-shift nurse.

"The mom's approach now is support to the max. The father has more conflict. He is very concerned for the suffering of the baby. They admit there is disagreement and that they are at each other's throats. They asked for counseling. We were able to refer. The baby is very responsive, and this is a particular curse for the family."

The father had a history of heavy drug abuse but was believed to have been drug free since he had been with his current wife. His health insurance was reaching its limit. In addition, he had been injured at work a few weeks earlier and was running out of disability insurance. The mother had begun to have migraine headaches. She was looking for work.

"We have the responsibility for a decision," committee chairman Dr. Ariagno said. "Our choices are, one, removal of intensive care, allowing the child to die, versus two, taking the approach that I think of as research—to see if nutrition and somatic growth bring any improvement in the lung function. We could reevaluate in six months, again in another six months. Anything else would be unfair to the family and the baby.

"I'm inclined to take the first approach," he said. "He is interesting. If he were a lab subject I would like to study him for the next year. But there is a minimum chance that he would survive." His description of the second alternative clearly showed that he considered it inhumane.

"How is number two different from what has been happening so far?" someone wanted to know.

"We waited for growth. Now more time and more investment by all would be involved."

Dr. Stevenson spoke. "I believe that when there is a chink of light to go for, go for it. There is already evidence of lung damage [from the respirator]. Based on the information so far, I believe there is no chance the baby will survive long term. There is no question that he would survive for a while. That is unfair. We are now embarked on an injurious mode." He recommended that mechanical ventilation be stopped, that the baby be fed and given oxygen, with the expectation that he would die. "We would tell the parents that he would die within minutes. But if the parents are not inclined to accept this, I would be inclined to proceed [to the second alternative]."

"For the mother, it is a matter of information and education," Dr. Ariagno said.

"We would need to reinforce what you just said, that treatment now is harmful," said the social worker. "But we need institutional agreement."

"In case there is a leak—the kind that people are always talking about," said one of the physicians, reminding the group that every decision to discontinue life support can explode into controversy, as the Baby Jane Doe decision did.

The hospital administrator said she agreed with the choice to discontinue. So did others. The nurses had been among the first to advocate letting this baby go.

"We would be switching, then, from an intensive care mode to a hospice mode," said Kathy Petersen, nailing down the consensus. "Yes," said Dr. Ariagno. "But this is not to be discussed. The decision is not yet made; it is still evolving, until the parents agree."

"Anyone disagree?" asked Petersen. Nobody did. It was policy that if anyone wanted to continue treatment in a case being considered, that would be done.

Josh's parents already knew, though nobody had told them in so many words, that the end was coming. They had told one of the staff that they wanted no bad news on Friday, the day after the meeting, because that was the father's birthday. The nurses made a birthday card with Josh's footprint on it.

On Saturday, one of the nurses called the parents and asked them to come in. Both attending physicians talked with them. They were careful to make clear that by agreeing to withdrawal of mechanical ventilation, the parents were not allowing their baby to die, that further attempts at therapy would only cause the baby more suffering without helping him to survive.

The parents were prepared for what they heard. They were aware of their child's suffering and ready to see it end right away. But after a moment's reflection, they decided to delay, so they could say good-bye in a more ceremonial way.

The father went to buy a new outfit for the baby, then to gather his parents and in-laws. Charlene Canger arranged for a $100 contribution for the funeral. At 5:00 P.M., the baby's parents, grandparents, and a priest gathered around his bed. The priest conducted a service. Then the family went into the small room adjacent to the nursery, where parents sometimes spent the night. Petersen and one of the primary nurses joined them. As the father of an infant the same age as Josh, Dr. Stevenson found his task especially difficult. As he removed the endotracheal tube that had kept Josh alive since his birth, tears flowed down his cheeks. He carried the infant to his parents.

Josh Patrick expired immediately. He tried to breathe for about a minute, then became unconscious. "One minute he was pink and cooing, responding. Two minutes later he was dead," Petersen said. "Before this I knew intellectually that technology keeps people alive. But I had never seen it so clearly. You can't help but grieve," she reflected. "But the way it was all done—the meeting, the whole process—provided closure for me, support for the parents and the staff. I had a rough week after that, but I had a foundation for understanding."

The day-shift primary nurse chose not to be present at the death, fearing she might be invading the family's privacy. So she did not have that closure, and, as she came back to the nursery the next morning, she had a flash of fear: What if he hadn't died? What then? But even as she thought this, she knew differently. Another baby occupied the spot where Josh had been.

Of course the control over the timing and mode of death is a matter of degree, no less so than control over who survives under intensive care. Some babies linger, then suddenly collapse and nothing more can be done. Sometimes it is not possible to wait until the family can be summoned. The baby just goes. But frequently a baby can be sustained for a few hours or a day or two, and physicians do that when they believe the family would benefit. It is at this point more than in any other aspect of their practice that physicians might be said to be playing God.

Once, a decision was made to keep a dying infant alive till morning because, in a doctor's opinion, her mother would find the death emotionally easier to accept then. The baby was prepared in the evening by being taken off Pavulon, so the mother could feel her move as she held her for the last time. But when the baby began to fail after midnight, the physician in charge ordered that she be reparalyzed, to conserve her remaining energy so she might survive a few more hours, to die in the morning as scheduled. Other aggressive interventions were also continued. A tube was pushed through her chest wall to release some of the air that had accumulated in her chest cavity because of leakage from the lungs. When, despite it, the chest began to fill again, a second tube was proposed.

Some of the baby's caretakers thought all this amounted to needless suffering for the baby. An intern rebelled at the proposal for a second chest tube. "I just said I won't do it," she said. "I felt that the child had suffered a lot of pain and damage and that was enough. I could not stand to do anything more to her. And I thought the reason for delaying was silly. The mother was there in the hospital and *her* suffering was so intense that I thought it did not really matter what time of day it was."

The resident relayed the intern's views to the attending physician, who suggested morphine and consulted with the head nurse for a further opinion. The second chest tube was not inserted. The baby lasted till morning and died in her mother's presence.

On another night, a death was delayed overnight to avoid its occurrence on the parents' anniversary. The young doctor in charge of that baby during the last hours said she understood her senior colleagues' reasoning, "but I hated that night so much because all through it, practically, I sat by that baby's bed as we did everything we know how to do to keep her alive when she was trying so hard to die. And then the next morning, [the attending] came in and pulled the tube. Just like that. It seems so unfair."

The structure and operation of the nursery, and the nature of intensive care, do not always allow for the kind of orchestrated death that was arranged for Josh Patrick. Often parents are saying their last good-bye amid all the daily bustle. While their child is dying, another parent might be nursing her recovering infant a few feet away.

169

"It must be hard for parents, everything just going on when they feel the world should stop," remarked Dr. Stevenson, pausing for a moment at the nursery door toward the end of a particularly difficult day: three infants had died. "They hear people talking, laughing. Everything just continues. We're used to going from one thing to another. For them it must be terrible."

As he spoke, three people with weatherbeaten faces and rough hands were just leaving the nursery. Farmworkers from the South, they were parents and a relative who had just lost their baby. The infant had been home only five days when he went into respiratory failure; he died shortly after arrival at the hospital.

Two days later, the parents returned for the body, which had been held for autopsy. They walked down the gleaming hospital hall and out through the glass doors, country people in an alien place. The father was wearing jeans, a checked shirt, boots and an old brown felt hat. He carried his baby's body in a box, on which was printed "Disposable Grad-U-Feed."

When death is held at bay by technological intervention, someone must be responsible for recognizing when to allow death to come, and for acting on this recognition. This duty goes against the grain of people who are dedicated to saving lives. According to an old French proverb, the physician's job is to cure sometimes, to relieve often, and to comfort always. "This paradigm of the physician has been replaced in our century with the paradigm of the physician as unyielding foe of death," said Dr. William Benitz. "Personally, I think that is an inappropriate role model. Nonetheless, it is the one that is pursued by many physicians in their practice. It reflects a value that is firmly ingrained from society and premedical and medical education, and it is difficult to change to something more balanced."

In light of this cultural attitude, it is natural that physicians are sometimes unable to cope with the responsibility for positive action to allow death—even when continued treatment only prolongs the process of dying. The consequence is needless suffering by families and children, and futile expenditures of medical resources.

A case in point was John Noler, born with a rare condition called holoprosencephaly. Most of his midbrain was missing and he was having frequent seizures. He had only one nostril and, because newborns cannot breathe through their mouths, would have died at birth had not somebody put a tube down his esophagus, allowing for more effective ventilation.

The baby, with tube already inserted, had been sent to Stanford from a community hospital several towns away, ostensibly for diagnostic purposes. The referring physician had said he wanted his diagnosis confirmed. It was. The defect was fatal and the baby was sure to die soon. He would have expired at birth had the tube not been inserted. If it was removed after he began to breathe through his mouth, the process might take somewhat longer. He might even live for as long as a year, then succumb to pneumonia or die by aspiration of food. In any case, there was nothing an intensive care nursery could do to help him.

Stanford officials tried to return the baby to the hospital he had come from, but that institution would not take him back, claiming it lacked the staff required for his care. No other unit or facility would accept him. So the baby stayed in the ICN for several weeks, where he was fed intravenously and attached to a heart and respiration monitor. At rounds he was usually passed by. His presence was depressing to nurses, doctors, and to visiting parents. One afternoon the attending inquired why he was on the monitor and, getting no answer, ordered the machine removed. But this did not mean that he would have been allowed to expire if his breathing or heart had stopped. He would automatically have been resuscitated, because for some weeks nobody wrote a no code order. This baby was dying and could not be saved. Only a small tube was delaying the inevitable. Why did nobody remove the tube? doctors were asked when John Noler had spent more than two weeks in the ICN.

In theory, starting mechanical life support does not commit physicians to continuing. But in practice, a distinction is often made. In the opinion of one of the residents, taking out the tube would have been tantamount to putting a pillow over the baby's head. "What gives you the right to play God and discontinue someone's life support?" she asked.

The attending thought that, on the contrary, the responsible act would have been to remove the tube once the diagnosis was confirmed. However, the baby had arrived before he assumed charge of the nursery and he was just inheriting the situation. He made plans to speak to the parents, who seemed confused. Since the baby was alive, although they had been told weeks ago that his condition was fatal, their hopes had unfortunately been raised. The parents were poor, with little schooling.

The preceding attending, who had accepted the referral of the baby, was asked why the tube was not removed after the hopelessness of the baby's condition was established. He replied that the responsibility for removing it was the referring physician's. "Our charge was to obtain the information for the private physician and the family regarding the baby's potential and what might be an appropriate way to handle the problem," he said. He thought the referring physician should counsel the parents further. He also advised against sending the baby home, because the emotional and practical burden of his care would be overwhelming to the parents and their six-year-old daughter.

But in the end, John Noler did go home. A visiting nurse called on the family several times. She was impressed with the excellent care his mother gave him, spending "twenty hours a day" with the baby. She observed that the father, who was unemployed and at home, was not supportive, and that the six-year-old sister was troubled. She slept in the same room with the infant, who continued to have frequent seizures.

During the ensuing days, the family situation worsened. The mother did not sleep. She never left the house. The six-year-old began to have stomachaches and headaches and stopped going to school. She clung to her mother and asked her repeatedly whether she loved her.

One night, about a month after he was taken home, the infant began to vomit and turn blue. He may have aspirated some of his vomit. The parents told the visiting nurse that the baby was asleep most of the following day. The nurse thought he was probably in a semi-coma. Then he started to breathe intermittently. But the parents, instead of allowing the baby's suffering to end, rushed him to the community hospital where he was born. There, at their request, he was resuscitated. Twenty-four hours later, when his breathing again began to fail, he was at last allowed to pass on.

Thus, because life support was begun but not withdrawn after it was obvious that the baby could not survive, the infant's dying was artificially prolonged. Lacking philosophical or religious guidelines for the situation, the physicians and the parents became entrapped by a simple life-support device that had been meant only as a temporary measure. The consequences for the family were devastating: at last report, the parents were reported to be separating. The costs of care were borne by the public, through MediCal, the state medical aid program.

Why was this death deferred? The prevailing legal and social climate may have been a factor. Government regulations, malpractice suits, advocates of extreme aggressiveness in the use of technology, may have affected the doctors' judgment. But in this case, the baby was indubitably born dying and therefore completely within range of those permitted to die under the Baby Doe regulations. No court or advocate could possibly have contested withdrawal of the death-deferring tube.

As one ICN staff member, a veteran observer of decision making, saw it, the delay could be explained only by what she called gut-level fear. "Everyone is afraid—afraid to take a baby to die," she said. "It's not fear of malpractice suits or anything like that. It's the bottom line: nobody wants to be around a dying baby."

The cultural rejection of death is the background against which the moral dilemmas of modern medicine manifest themselves. Lately, a shift toward a more accepting attitude has begun, evidenced in the establishment of hospices and programs to help the dying and the publication of numerous books about death as the last stage of life. The process of grief has been studied as a process of personal growth.

For parents of marginally viable newborns, perhaps the most overwhelming sorrow comes with the death of a child who lives long enough to become known and loved as an individual and a part of the family, then succumbs. Such a child was Arthur Tuttle, who survived for three years with the help of supplementary oxygen but never outgrew his chronic lung disease.

More than three years after his death, Alice Tuttle, the child's mother, still could not talk about Arthur without crying. She no longer visited the grave daily—she went only about once a week—but Arthur was on her mind much of the time. She saw his features in his twin, Martin, and she worried excessively about the new baby, Thomas, who was, thank God, robust. As she watched him sleep and listened to his breathing, she remembered how she used to sit for hours listening to Arthur's breathing, "so fast, or else so shallow and distended." She checked on Thomas more than she really needed to do.

The surviving twin was also overanxious because of what he remembered. At night he sometimes called to her, "Mommy, Mommy, Thomas isn't breathing." She would come in and reassure him that the baby was fine, that he was merely sleeping.

Then she would stroke Martin's head and pray that he might outgrow the fears that were the residue of those three years.

The whole family paid a heavy price for the prolonged and futile effort to keep Arthur alive. They lived, day by day, between home and the hospital. The baby's father, Marshall Tuttle, was compelled to change jobs twice for the sake of an insurance policy that would cover a bill that went far past the half-million-dollar mark. His childhood asthma returned, and he himself needed the vaporizer that used to help keep Arthur's airways clear.

Alice would not wish what she went through on anyone, but Arthur is so deep a part of her life now that she cannot imagine herself not having known him. "I'm not bitter anymore," she said. "I know there is a reason why he lived. I asked God, 'If you kept him alive for three years, why did you take him away?' But I know his life had a purpose and he accomplished that purpose. There were times when I thought we were being selfish in trying to hold him. He was already so tired; his body was so tired."

She has a poem Dr. Ariagno wrote for Arthur on his second birthday:

> . . . reaching, deeply reaching, and you are only two
> Little need discussing what we can and cannot do—
> Many tears shed over that . . .

Arthur is one of the babies Dr. Ariagno remembers when he talks about the need for more research to help improve the outcome for neonatal intensive care survivors and to help understanding catch up with the available technology.

They were not the smallest of premature infants, but they were very sick. Martin was 2.9 pounds at birth, Arthur 2.14. Both had suffered respiratory distress at birth in a community hospital and were transferred to Stanford, where they were hit by a virus infection. Martin recovered in two months and went home. Although he had some neurological and other deficits that would become apparent later, he seemed fine at the time. But Arthur's lungs deteriorated into bronchopulmonary dysplasia. He stayed on the respirator much longer than his brother and, when he finally was pronounced ready to go home, was still attached to an oxygen supply. Oxygen was blown past his nostrils through a tube taped to his cheeks.

As Arthur grew older and became mobile, the tube was extended, so he could move around in his room. But he could go without the supplemental oxygen for only a short time and often, even with it, he would gasp and turn blue and be rushed back to the hospital. His lungs were severely damaged.

Alice spent much of her time in those three years at the Stanford hospital, first in the intensive care nursery, then in the pediatrics ward, then in Children's Hospital. Arthur never managed to stay home more than three months at a time. Wherever he was, the family's whole life revolved around him.

"They never promised me anything," said Alice Tuttle. "Always they said, 'We don't know.' But what I never expected was that he would come home and not get off the oxygen. His need for it increased. He was in and out of the hospital. Stanford was his second home. He was hurting. I had to tell him, 'I'm sorry, Arthur. It hurts me that you are hurting.' And he would look up to me in his own way: 'Mommy, why?'"

Arthur died at the hospital on Valentine's Day 1981, just as his family was preparing to go visit him. "He was supposed to go home the next day," said his mother. "But his heart was so weak that he couldn't go on anymore.

"After that I got pregnant again right away and miscarried. Twice. The third time I was very apprehensive. I wanted to prove I could have a normal baby. I kept praying, 'Please God, don't let it be a preemie this time.' But the baby came out healthy, very red, and he cried right away. He had so much hair. His nails and his lips were so red. Arthur was blue. And Martin was very red, with white film. But this baby, Thomas, he was a term baby, he was thirty-eight weeks. Praise God, he is now almost eleven weeks old."

As a result of her experience, Alice Tuttle decided she would like to resume the nurse's training she began in the Philippines. But she would wait until later. Right now not only the new baby but also Martin had special need of her. He had been found to be somewhat behind his age level in mental development and, in addition, was recently discovered to be suffering from hearing impairment in both ears. He was hospitalized three times for an operation to implant a tube in the middle ear to facilitate drainage. The tube fell out twice. Alice hoped that this time it would stay. Martin was afraid of the hospital—afraid he might die there, as his brother had.

Alice was trying to focus her mind on the children who were alive and needed her, but she said, "I never knew what suffering was until I had Arthur. It's a hurt so deep I cannot explain it and it does not get less."

Eventually, grief can be transformed into a heightened awareness and a commitment to life. Like the priest who learned about conscious dying in Alaska, Ellen Miles, who lost a two-month-old daughter, came to see her child's brief life and her death, together, as a gift.

Mrs. Miles is a respiratory therapist at Stanford Medical Center, working with newborns, older children, and adults. One afternoon, after finishing her day's work in the pediatrics ward, she sat on a sunny deck of the hospital and told about Sarah. She spoke calmly and thoughtfully. The grief that was still tearing at Alice Tuttle had, in Ellen Miles, matured into affirmation.

"I was thirty-five, in my last quarter of respiratory therapy school, when my birth control failed. I was concerned because I was taking a medication for a condition I had, but a doctor told me it would not be a problem. It was, though. I had polyhydramnios." An excessive amount of amniotic fluid accumulated in her uterus, so much that her weight rose suddenly and enormously.

"I was forced to leave school and spend the last three months of my pregnancy in hospital bed rest, moving every fifteen minutes so circulation to my heart would not be compromised. This was tough on my family. My husband was wonderful, cooking and caring for the children, who were then seven and ten. For weeks I could not see them because the hospital had a rule of no children under twelve. Finally, the doctor made an exception because I was in there so long." The children became withdrawn; their grades dropped. The younger one began to have trouble in school.

A glucose test showed that Ellen had gestational diabetes. "Its effect on the baby was an irreparable cardiac defect. The effect of the drug I had been taking was facial abnormalities—low-set ears, wide-set eyes, small fingernail beds."

The delivery was traumatic. The doctors had assumed that the baby was small, about five pounds. In fact she was nine pounds five ounces, too big for Ellen to deliver vaginally without help.

"When I went into labor there was a full moon and fifteen women were in four delivery rooms. The doctors were extremely busy. Had they decided to do a C-section, there would have been no place to do it. My cardiac circulation was too stressed for transportation to another hospital. So a doctor pulled, three nurses pushed. She was born with fractured ribs and severe intercranial bleeding from being wedged a long time in the birth canal with the cord compressed.

"A lot could have been done differently, I suppose, but nothing that would have kept her alive. With a C-section she still would have had the cardiac defect, a valve problem that was inoperable. They resuscitated her, gave her oxygen, transferred her to the University of California Medical Center in San Francisco, put in a cardiac catheter. Eventually we were told we could take her home and just give her medications. They never tell you she will die—because they never know. There are miracles. But I knew, basically, that she would not make it past two years, though nobody actually said so.

"We had her for ten days, and they were the true gift of having Sarah—the breast-feeding, sleeping in bed together, sharing normal baby experiences that are joyful. I realize, looking back on it now, that it was difficult. But at the time I was racing to get as much of my Sarah as I was going to get and they were wonderful days.

"On the tenth day she started having increased respiration problems. Her heart started beating very fast. We took her in and she was put on oxygen. And suddenly I was sitting there focusing on the monitor. I noticed her heart rhythm had dropped abnormally and knew she was not going to come back.

"They resuscitated her for over an hour. We kept waiting. At the end all they had to offer was, did I want to hold her? I did. I had read all the books on death and dying in school and I realized the importance of that last contact.

"She was so warm. Often you hear how babies that come in so sick are beautiful as they die. At birth she had been extremely puffy. Now she had lost a lot of that weight, she was five pounds, with big eyes, dark hair, long eyelashes. She was beautiful. I said, 'Are you sure she is not alive?' She was pink, she was warm. I asked the nurse to tell my husband to come in, it was okay. He did and he held her and he thanked me later. Sarah's nurse came in. She also needed to say good-bye.

"After that my husband was very generous, and I decided to be generous to myself. I took a year and a half to be home, to be a mom—struggling to go by baby stores without breaking down. After that I realized that Sarah had been an occurrence in our life that brought us all closer together as a family, though we already had been close. She was the only child my husband and I had together. He was my second husband; we married when my other children were very young. He said to me, 'Don't ever say, I wish I could give you a baby. We had a baby. She was special and she was loved. It's just that she lived a very short time.'

"I think this was an experience that helped me not only for myself but for the work that I do," said Ellen Miles. "When Sarah died, it was the right time. It was her time to die."

Dr. Elisabeth Kübler-Ross, who has spent years working with dying children, has written, "If we can learn to view death from a different perspective, to reintroduce it into our lives so that it comes not as a dreaded stranger but as an expected companion to our life, then we can also learn to live our lives with meaning—with full appreciation of our finiteness, of the limits on our time here."[3]

That attitude is a prerequisite for the conscious choices about dying that medical technology requires physicians, parents, and society at large to make. As these stories from one intensive care center show, a child's death can also be a gift of life. It has been the experience of doctors, as well as parents, that sometimes, after a child dies with respectful recognition, they feel a lightness of spirit and come away uplifted.

Part Three
Isolettes in the
Modern World

CHAPTER EIGHT

The Limits of Choice—

Baby Doe to Baby Fae

Since April 30, 1982, the federal government has been a shadowy participant in decision making about borderline-viable infants. On that date, President Ronald Reagan moved to take choice on this issue out of physicians' hands. He issued an order that, in effect, required that very premature, very damaged, or very sick newborns be treated as aggressively as infants without serious handicaps. Neither doctors nor parents were to have any alternative. This unprecedented presidential intervention into life-and-death choices at the threshold of birth came in response to the urging of pro-life and disability groups, in the midst of a nationwide controversy about an infant known as Baby Doe.

Baby Doe was born in Bloomington, Indiana, on April 9, 1982, with Down's syndrome and other abnormalities. He died six days later after his parents, with the support of their obstetrician, withheld their consent for surgery that would probably have continued his life, but would not have reversed the mental retardation associated with Down's syndrome. His story drew national publicity to a controversy that had, until then, been under way primarily in the pages of medical and philosophical journals, among religious groups, and among medical practitioners. It became a barometer of public opinion.

Reagan's election to the presidency had marked a turning away from the liberal tradition and the ascendance of the right-to-life movement from the status of an extremist fringe group to a position of considerable power. The president had appointed as the surgeon general Dr. C. Everett Koop, a pediatric surgeon who was an uncompromising advocate of life-at-any-cost for fetuses and newborns. He had spoken and written widely and passionately on the right-to-life issue.

At one time, in a booklet, *The Right to Live; The Right to Die* (1976), he stated that he had accepted abortion in some "hard" cases out of "Christian compassion." But then he had met a nurse who told him she would expect her own daughter to carry to term a pregnancy resulting from rape. So he had ruled out exceptions.

In that same booklet, Dr. Koop also argued for heroic measures with extremely damaged newborns, backing his case with a fundamentalist interpretation of the Bible and with testimonials, rather than with factual evidence. He viewed as treatable even an infant born with "no rectum, whose bladder is inside out, whose abdominal organs are out in his umbilical cord, and who has a cleft spine with an opening in his back so you can see his spinal cord," with legs "in such a position that his feet lie most comfortably next to his ears." Dr. Koop asserted that every one of those defects was "correctable." In a footnote he added, "I treated a boy who had half of these things plus a few others. He has had more than twenty-five operations. I see him and his family in the community about once a week. They are a great family and consider the boy and his problems to be the best experience life has offered them. The boy is a delight." No particulars are given: what the boy's condition is, what his life is like, what his care requires.[1]

Further along, Dr. Koop makes the startling statement that "studies on handicapped children have indicated that their frustrations are no greater than those experienced by perfectly normal children." He offers no references or documentation, merely the avowal, "To this latter fact I can attest."[2]

The appointment of a man with such attitudes as the chief medical officer of the United States would have been inconceivable a decade earlier. But the country's moral climate had changed radically since then. Individual rights won during the previous decades were being eroded. Tolerance for diversity had diminished, as had concern about social injustice. The economy was going through wrenching changes, and many people felt that traditional values somehow had to be shored up.

The right-to-life movement had grown along with fundamentalist Christian groups and had helped to elect President Reagan. One of the catalysts was the fear generated by the personal liberation movements, particularly the women's movement. The leading women's rights activists had framed their struggle in terms of power and posed the issue of abortion as one of "reproductive freedom" and "body sovereignty." These terms failed to acknowledge the continuum and interconnectedness of life and the acute dilemma that abortion represents for most women. Intent on securing for women the right to end an unwanted pregnancy, leading activists used rhetoric that oversimpified the issue. Had there been, instead of bumper stickers defending abortion, new systems of sisterly support for women who took this difficult option, perhaps the opposition movement, which proclaimed that the fetus had a right to life at any cost, would not have acquired so much power.

Of course, the women's movement was only one factor in the rise of the anti-abortion movement, which, it should be noted, has men rather than women in many leadership roles. Nor was the women's rights movement monolithic. Grace Paley, the writer, once envisioned herself and her friends walking behind three banners: one for choice on abortion, one for peace, and the third reading, "Joy to the child, our gift and our friend." But the lack of that kind of vision among the most audible voices during the height of the women's movement's strength, in the 1970s, left an opening for its opponents to declare themselves the champions of abandoned infants, the defenders of families, and to call themselves pro-life.

On closer inspection, it was obvious that *life* was defined in the narrowest of terms, and the defense of the family was largely rhetoric. A 1984 analysis of the voting record of sixty pro-life and sixty pro-choice national legislators, conducted by Catholics for a Free Choice, found that anti-choice legislators tended to oppose other bills aiming to help children and families (by providing child-care, nutritional, and other support), while pro-choice senators and congressmen tended to vote in favor of these bills. The concern of anti-abortionists with the prevention of fetal and newborn deaths at any cost did not lead to support of other children's needs. (Curiously, many life-at-any-cost champions also favor capital punishment, seeing no contradiction.)

If feminists, in the intensity of the fight for more power, temporarily failed to consider women's symbiosis with children, the pro-life groups forgot it because of their fixation on embryo and fetus. Dr. Koop, for instance, after pointing out that *fetus* is a medical term that can be used to sanitize the abortion issue, uses *unborn baby* and *uterus* in the same sentence, choosing the distancing of the Latin term over the flesh-and-blood word *womb*.[3]

Dr. Bernard Nathanson, an anti-abortionist known for his dubious abortion documentary, *The Silent Scream*, was quoted in a *Newsweek* article as saying, "With the aid of technology, we stripped away the walls of the abdomen and looked into the womb."[4] The violence of the image is chilling. The woman has ceased to exist as a person.

Beneath the abortion issue, which pitted women's rights activists against fundamentalist Christians and other pro-lifers, lay a deeper unease about the consequences of progress in control over reproduction. The abortion issue is inseparable from neonatology because birth has ceased to be a meaningful dividing line between baby and fetus in the context of the modern hospital. New procedures allow many birth defects to be detected early enough for abortion. But neonatology kept pushing back the threshold of viability and late abortions came disquietingly close to the age at which a fetus/baby can survive with intensive care. Occasionally, a fetus emerged alive from a late abortion and was rushed to the intensive care nursery. Some doctors and nurses consequently refused to participate in late abortions, not on traditional religious grounds but because they felt they were coming too close to infanticide. This situation was one of the moral anomalies created by rapid advances in obstetrics, perinatology, and neonatology. The law was unable to keep up with new developments in the modern medical center; neither could traditional moral norms. It is worth noting, for instance, that both Baby Doe and Baby Jane Doe could have been legally aborted late during gestation without stirring up any kind of trouble.

All this created havoc with traditional ways of thinking about birth. In addition, there were the rapid innovations in artificial conception. Women had an unprecedented degree of choice, not only in whether to bear a baby but also when and how and what kind of baby. Previously infertile women managed—usually at great expense—to bear children with the help of in vitro fertilization, embryo transplants, and other methods. Lesbian women were achieving pregnancy with sperm donated by anonymous homosexual men, which was implanted with turkey basters. Fertilization was becoming a big business. In 1982, about one million women received medical advice or treatment for infertility, while 1.5 million pregnancies, a fourth of the total, ended in abortion. Society seemed to be moving toward a future of custom-made babies.

The infant who was to become known as Baby Doe was born into this environment of increasing intervention in the process of life's beginnings and, within days, became front-page news and the subject of intense medical, legal, and ethical debate. The infant of two former schoolteachers who had two other children, he was asphyxiated at birth, resuscitated with oxygen, and then found to have signs of Down's syndrome and a malformation called esophageal atresia with tracheoesophageal fistula. That is, his esophagus had failed to develop normally, ending in a blind pouch rather than serving as a channel between throat and stomach. The stomach end of the interrupted esophagus linked directly to the windpipe, so that stomach juices backed up and could eventually digest the lungs. Breathing would also be impeded by the baby's inability to get rid of mucus. His first Apgar score was a low 2 out of a possible 10.

The obstetrician gave the parents a choice: they could permit the baby to be transported to a hospital forty miles away, where the surgery to save his life would be performed. Such surgery usually involves considerable pain and may have to be followed by more surgery in the years to come, he told them. It would repair the esophagus but do nothing about the retardation accompanying Down's syndrome. The other route, he told the parents, was to withhold consent for the surgery, in which case the infant would almost certainly die of pneumonia in a few days. The parents opted for nontreatment. The baby was to be sedated and kept comfortable until he expired.[5]

The physician who had offered the parents the choice believed that the baby, and his family, would be better off if he died, because his existence could be no more than minimal. But the dying took six days, was difficult, and caused a disturbance beyond expectations.

Other physicians sharply opposed the obstetrician's offering nontreatment to the family. Nurses rebelled and asked that the infant be moved from the nursery into a private room. Two nurses who had to care for the baby were extremely distressed and later sought psychotherapy. Hospital officials, knowing that, legally, they were sitting on a powder keg, asked a Monroe County superior judge for an opinion. The judge ruled that since there were two medical opinions, the parents had the right to choose. Then, after right-to-lifers heard of the case and attacked him, the judge asked the county public welfare department's child protection committee to review the decision. It was upheld.

But the issue was then picked up by county prosecutors who disagreed with the decision and proceeded to seek a court order to perform the surgery. They met with no success. The Indiana Supreme Court refused to hear the case. The baby died while the prosecutors were en route to Washington to appeal to the Supreme Court. By this time the story was big news, generating much emotion nationwide.

Right-to-lifers and advocate groups for the disabled turned to the White House, urging President Reagan to take action. He responded by ordering Richard Schweiker, then secretary of Health and Human Services (HHS), to notify health care providers receiving federal funds that, under Section 504 of the Rehabilitation Act of 1973, they risked losing those funds if they withheld nourishment or treatment from disabled newborns. The law forbids withholding from the handicapped, simply because of the handicap, any benefit or service that would ordinarily be provided to people without handicaps. It has been used effectively to assure access to public facilities for people in wheelchairs by provision of ramps and other aids. It had never been used to affect physicians' actions with respect to newborns. Reagan declared, "Our nation's commitment to equal protection of the law will have little meaning if we deny such protection to those who have not been blessed with the same physical or mental gifts we too often take for granted."

HHS sent the requested notice, signed by Betty Lou Dotson, then director of the Office of Civil Rights, to the administrators of sixty-eight hundred hospitals nationwide. Then, on March 2, 1983, came another HHS directive, an "interim final rule." In addition to the previous notice, which became known as the Baby Doe regulations, the rule required that warning signs be posted in delivery rooms, nurseries, intensive care nurseries, and pediatrics units, to read as follows: "Discriminatory failure to feed and care for handicapped infants in this facility is prohibited by federal law. Failure to feed and care for infants may also violate the criminal and civil laws of your state." The notice was also to inform the public of the existence of a toll-free hot line in Washington, where someone was ready, twenty-four hours a day, to hear reports about allegedly mistreated infants.

On March 18, four days before these regulations were to become effective, a suit was filed in U.S. District Court, by the American Academy of Pediatrics and several other medical groups, against HHS and its new secretary, Margaret Heckler. On April 18, Justice Gerhard Gesell found that the new rule violated procedural requirements for advance notice and public comment, that it was "arbitrary and capricious, and virtually without meaning beyond its intrinsic *in terrorem* effect." He declared it invalid. New proposed regulations were issued July 5, 1983, allowing sixty days for public comment. They bore the personal imprint of Dr. Koop.

"Strangely, the rules make no mention of the suffering of severely handicapped newborns," observed Dr. Marcia Angell in the *New England Journal of Medicine* of September 15. "Instead they express the concern that a physician might decide that 'a person is not worthy of treatment.' This wording is mischievous in its implication. The issue in neonatal intensive-care units is *not* one of 'worthiness' but one of future suffering. Do we have the right to inflict a life of suffering on a helpless newborn just because we have the technology to do so and despite the fact that we ourselves would have the legal right to reject such a life?"[6]

After the period allowed for comment had ended and before the final rules were adopted, another national debate flared up about a defective infant, dramatizing Dr. Angell's point. The child, who was to become known as Baby Jane Doe, was born October 11, 1983, in St. Charles Hospital, Port Jefferson, New York, and transferred to the neonatal intensive care unit in University Hospital, State University of New York at Stony Brook. She was so damaged that there was no doubt she was destined only for lifelong institutional care.

The diagnosis showed a large lumbosacral myelomeningocele, microencephaly, hydrocephalus, and other birth defects, meaning that part of the baby's spinal cord was abnormally developed and exposed; she was unable to move her lower extremities and did not seem to have sensation below her lower trunk; her head was abnormally tiny, and fluid was pressing on her brain. It was apparent that she would have no control over her bladder or bowels. She was almost certainly brain-damaged and would suffer from severe mental retardation. When the parents learned of these defects, and were told that there were probably others that had not been detected, they decided against surgery to close the exposed spinal cord. They did so after consulting with physicians, nurses, relatives, religious advisers, and a social worker. The baby was fed, placed in an incubator, and sterile dressings were applied.

When right-to-lifers learned that the parents had declined surgical intervention, they went to court to force them to accept it. The proceedings that followed were to last ten months as the physicians and the hospital fought right-to-life groups and the Reagan administration. The parents would endure not only the tragedy of their child but national publicity as well.

A right-to-life attorney, Lawrence Washburn, who lived in Vermont and had never seen the baby or the parents, sought and obtained court appointment of a guardian ad litem, who would have the power to consent to the surgery, transfer the baby to another hospital, and examine the records. Justice Frank DeLuca of the New York State Supreme Court (the court of first instance in that state) acted without notification to hospital or parents.

On October 18, 1983 the guardian visited the hospital and reported to the court that he was satisfied that the infant was receiving adequate medical care and attention. He noted that the issue was whether additional treatment was possible within the standards of care, and, if so, whether the court should order it despite the parents' wishes.

The same day, Gene Curran, a representative of the American Life Lobby, sent a telegram to HHS in Washington, alerting the department to the case and asking them to "act immediately."

HHS responded by filing a complaint with the Suffolk County Department of Child Protective Services, alleging neglect. The agency, which had been created by federal law specifically to investigate suspected instances of child abuse and neglect, looked into the case and found the complaint to have been unfounded.

The following day, hearings began in the New York State Supreme Court before Justice Melvyn Tanenbaum. Dr. George Newman, the neurologist who had been caring for the baby, testified about her condition.

He said, "On the basis of the combinations of the malformations that are present in this child, she is not likely to ever achieve any meaningful interaction with her environment, nor ever to achieve any interpersonal relationships, the very qualities that we consider human, . . . she is capable of experiencing pain. . . . As I think she has only limited ability to experience comfort, and primarily an ability to experience pain, to perform this surgery would increase the total pain that the child would experience."[7]

He estimated that with surgery she could live twenty years; without it she would almost certainly die within two.

In a later interview with a *Newsday* reporter, Dr. Albert Butler, chief of neurosurgery at the Stony Brook hospital, saw a slightly less grim possibility. He said the worst-case prognosis would be to live, lying in bed, unable to do anything, having seizures, while the best case would be a borderline-educable handicapped person. He said, however, that he would never advocate forcing parents to consent to surgery for their infant in such a situation.

Justice Tanenbaum found "that the infant is in imminent danger, and that the infant has an independent right to survive: that right must be protected by the State acting in parens patriae."[8] He ordered that a neurosurgeon associated with the hospital perform the surgery and that the guardian ad litem be empowered to give the consent ordinarily granted by parents. After Judge Tanenbaum issued his decision, however, the court was notified that the baby had a fever of 102 degrees, which precluded surgery. Another justice granted a stay to the parents' attorney.

On October 20, in a unanimous decision, a five-judge panel of the appellate division of the state Supreme Court reversed the trial court. In its decision, the panel stressed that this case was different from the *Baby Doe* case, that "this is not a case where an infant is being deprived of medical treatment to achieve a quick and supposedly merciful death. Rather it is a situation where the parents have chosen one course of appropriate medical treatment over another. These concededly concerned and loving parents made an informed, intelligent, and reasonable determination based upon and supported by responsible medical authority. . . . [We] find the parents' determination to be in the best interest of the infant."[9]

Before the decision was announced, the HHS Office of Civil Rights began an investigation and demanded access to the baby's medical records and a meeting with her physicians at 10:00 A.M. the next day. The hospital refused. The federal government took its case to court and lost on February 23, 1984, at the Second Circuit U.S Court of Appeals. In a 2 to 1 decision, the court stated that a review of the legislative history had shown that Congress never contemplated that Section 504 of the Rehabilitation Act be applied to treatment decisions involving defective newborn infants.

Meanwhile, in mid-December, the spinal defect had closed spontaneously. The baby was treated with antibiotics for infection. A shunt was performed, with parental agreement, to ease the fluid buildup in her cranial cavity. She was discharged from the hospital at six months of age, to the care of her parents. At ten months, during a developmental test, her cognitive functioning was found to be in a low range, significantly less than normal for age. She was paraplegic and her sight was impaired.

In September 1984, Congress passed the Child Abuse Amendments of 1984, which established regulations on treatment of handicapped newborns as federal law. President Reagan signed the bill into law October 9, 1984. The event was scarcely noted by the media.

The law requires that all disabled infants, with only three exceptions, be afforded medically indicated treatment. The exceptions are somewhat ambiguously described. They are, first, those who are "chronically and irreversibly comatose," second, those for whom treatment would "merely prolong dying, not be effective in ameliorating or correcting all of the infant's life-threatening conditions, or otherwise be futile in terms of survival," and third, if the treatment would be "virtually futile in terms of survival" and "under such circumstances would be inhumane." The physician's "reasonable medical judgment" must be prudent, knowledgeable about the case and treatment possibilities with respect to medical conditions involved. "It is not to be based on subjective 'quality of life' or other abstract concepts."[10]

This last proviso requires an abrupt departure from the tradition of the decision-making process with very sick or damaged newborns, as it is described in *Deciding to Forego* [sic] *Life-Sustaining Treatment: Ethical, Medical, and Legal Issues in Treatment Decisions* (March 1983), the report of the President's Commission for the Study of Ethical Problems in Medicine and Biomedical and Behavioral Research. The commission, appointed by President Jimmy Carter, issued its report less than a month after the death of Baby Doe. It stated:

> In most circumstances, people agree on whether a proposed course of therapy is in the patient's best interest. Even with seriously ill newborns, quite often there is no issue—either a particular therapy

plainly offers net benefits, or no effective therapy is available. Sometimes, however, the right outcome will be unclear because the child's "best interests" are difficult to define.[11]

According to the commission, there are three categories of seriously ill newborns: those who would clearly benefit from aggressive therapy, those for whom it would clearly be futile, and ambiguous cases. But though such classification seems to make sense, it is by no means obvious what babies would belong in each category. The vast majority of infants in an ICN would be in the first—those who would benefit. The commission made a point of including Down's infants, stating that "the handicaps of Down's Syndrome, for example . . . do not justify failing to provide medically proven treatment, such as surgical correction of a blocked intestinal tract" but not dealing with the moral anomaly of a "therapeutic" abortion after Down's syndrome is discovered by amniocentesis.[12]

Angela Walker-Shaw was in the first category. But had she been born in a remote rural hospital instead of in a fully equipped and staffed medical center, she might not have been.

Preemies whose systems are too undeveloped to allow intubation and respiratory support are in the second category, as are preemies who might have a chance in a good ICN but are born too far away from one to be transported there in time. So, of course, are babies, like John Noler, born with an undeveloped brain, and babies, like Josh Patrick, with severe chest-wall deformity. Did Chris Lew belong in this category? The physicians at the hospital where he was born believed he did; the surgeons at Stanford did not. His death does not really settle the issue, for the surgeons thought the operation to repair his fatal defect had succeeded.

An infant does not necessarily remain in the same category. Maria de Jesús Rodriguez is a case in point. When the ethics committee decided that, parents willing, it would be acceptable to refrain from escalating treatment, it did so because its members saw no effective therapy available for her neurologic condition. But later, when it was decided that she should have heart surgery in the hope of helping her off the respirator, net benefits were envisioned. The surgery was successful, but her basically grim prospects were unchanged.

In the third category, when it is hard to define an infant's best interests, the ambiguity has traditionally made the decision making most difficult. The commission notes that neonatology "is too new a field to allow accurate predictions of which babies will survive and of the complications, handicaps, and potentials that the survivors might have."[13] Prognosis becomes easier the longer infants in the last category survive; however, each added week or month of survival also increases the possibility of inflicting harm on such infants, violating the principle *Primum non nocere*. The longer an infant lives, the more difficult it is to make decisions about withholding or withdrawing aggressive care. The story of Matthew Cordell is an excellent case in point.

Over the years, a consensus has emerged among ethicists and physicians, namely, that with respect to infants in the ambiguous category, parental considerations and societal provisions for support should be allowed to weigh more heavily than with infants in the other two categories. That is, if it is clear that an infant would benefit from aggressive therapy and that parents are opposed, their objections should be overruled, by means of a court injunction, if necessary. Likewise, if the physicians see no hope that an infant would benefit from treatment and the parents insist on it, their wishes should be followed only long enough to allow medical professionals to help them understand the futility of their demand. But if an infant has the potential for survival, although with profound disabilities—mental, physical, or both— as did Maria Rodriguez, then consideration should be given to what the parents and society would provide for the support of the infant.

It was this broad consensus that Dr. Anthony Shaw, a pediatric surgeon at the University of Virginia Medical Center, reflected and expressed in what he termed his "formula without numbers." In an article titled "Who Should Die and Who Should Decide?"[14] Shaw suggested the following formula: $QOL = NE \times (H + S)$, with QOL representing quality of life, NE a child's natural endowment, and H and S the contributions from home and society. A child with anencephaly (absence of all or a major part of the brain) would have a natural endowment of zero, whatever the home and society provided. A Down's syndrome child would have a higher NE. The figure for the quality of his life could rise or fall, depending on how much home and society contributed in care and support. According to Shaw, "If the family of a baby with Down's syndrome refused to care for it, and society's sole contribution is a crowded, filthy, understaffed warehouse, that infant's quality of life equals zero ($NE \times (O + O) = O$) just as surely as if it had been born an anencephalic."[15]

However, Shaw's formula is more useful in formulating policy than it is in clinical decision making, for the specific endowment of most newborns remains largely a matter of speculation. Statistical data can provide a basis for projecting outcome on the basis of probability, but each individual is a potential exception because each is unique. No formula exists to aid the physician, health care team, and parents with the most difficult choices. The Baby Doe regulations, in effect, decree that all infants in the ambiguous category be treated as though they were in the category of those for whom treatment is clearly beneficial. For some doctors, that law may be a rationale for setting qualms aside and treating everyone relentlessly. A well-known neonatologist has remarked that "some people in this country will hook a turnip up to a respirator, saying they are doing all they can to save this individual—for whom they have no treatment." But the law can be only an obstacle to those who seek to sort out available facts, in light of their perceptions, values, and the parents' wishes, and to select a course toward the child's best interest.

From a future perspective, the Baby Doe regulations will no doubt turn out to have been little more than one step in the long struggle with the ever-increasing moral quandaries besetting medical practice. They represent, among other things, a fumbling attempt to expand concern over these issues. They have had the effect, especially within hospitals, of escalating the national debate about newborn intensive care.

The degree of life-or-death choice being exercised in the nursery first came sharply to the medical community's attention in 1973, nine years before Baby Doe, with the publication of an article titled "Moral and Ethical Dilemmas in the Special-Care Nursery," in the *New England Journal of Medicine*. The authors, Raymond S. Duff, professor of pediatrics in the Yale University School of Medicine, and his associate, A. G. M. Campbell, who subsequently became professor of child health, University of Aberdeen, Scotland, described their policy of selective nontreatment of infants in the Yale-New Haven Hospital. During a period of thirty months, this nursery admitted 2171 infants. Of the 299 who died, 43 expired after medical treatment was withdrawn. All had serious defects, including multiple anomalies, chromosomal and cardiopulmonary problems, myelomeningocele (spina bifida). The outlook for all had been judged to be dismal or hopeless, and physicians, with the participation of parents, had made a decision to withdraw treatment. Drs. Duff and Campbell made a plea for allowing parents a choice when the effectiveness of treatment was in serious doubt.

In this same issue of the New England journal, Dr. Shaw described eight cases in which a decision to withdraw treatment was considered and proposed a system for thinking about such decisions.[16]

As neonatology advanced, more physicians went public with their moral dilemmas. In England, Dr. John Lorber, a pediatrician in the Children's Hospital, Western Bank, Sheffield, reported that in his experience, treating all infants born with spina bifida "resulted in massive suffering for the largest number in spite of massive cost to the community."[17] Between 1959 and 1968, 848 infants were treated in the Sheffield hospital. Half were still alive four to fourteen years later, but only six of these 424 survived with no handicap. Over 80 percent had severe physical disabilities; 17 percent had "moderate" ones. Conditions termed "moderate," however, included some that to most people would have been serious: absence of bladder or rectal sphincter control, hydrocephalus, and partial paralysis. The children were subjected to surgery repeatedly throughout their lives, Dr. Lorber reported, and they grew progressively stunted and deformed with age. It was much harder for parents to lose an older child than to have a disabled infant die at birth.

"As time went on and our experience increased, it became apparent that in spite of the progressively increasing survival rate the problems we created were greater than those we solved," Dr. Lorber later said.[18] As a result, he adopted a policy of nontreatment for infants born with the most severe cases of spina bifida.

Drs. Duff, Campbell, Shaw, and Lorber were ferociously attacked, accused of playing God and of killing infants. But what they had acknowledged openly was being practiced quietly in many hospitals. They had confronted an immensely troubling moral issue and compelled its further consideration.

The debate about the proper limits of treatment came at a time when physicians were losing the mantle of authority that had long screened their activities from the public. Patients were demanding to see their charts, to have procedures and medications explained, to be told of options in treatment. There was a great deal of interest in self-care and alternative forms of medicine, and widespread criticism of the medical profession. Malpractice suits proliferated, particularly against obstetricians, and the plaintiffs found sympathetic jurors.

In response, since 1980 almost every major hospital has either retained an ethicist as consultant or added one to its staff. More recently, in the wake of the new federal law, increasing numbers have also established ethics committees.

The ethicist is usually a philosopher, theologian, or one who has studied extensively in these disciplines and the related field of ethics. In a medical center, the ethicist's job is to help practitioners and researchers find their way through the moral issues that arise in the course of their work. He or she does this by applying analytic skills to sort out key elements that bear on decisions and to assure that they are considered. The activities of the ethicist usually include consultation on individual cases and on broader policy issues, teaching, and participation on ethics committees.

Some years ago, the Stanford medical center ethicist was invited by the resident on call in the pediatrics ward to help consider the case of a boy who had spent his entire two and a half years of life in the hospital, kept alive technologically although he had no hope of recovery. At birth, he had been diagnosed as having chronic, idiopathic, irritable bowel syndrome. An older sibling had died two years earlier of the same condition—untreatable, constant diarrhea that prevented him from absorbing food. Nasogastric tube feeding was out of the question, for nothing remained in the child's stomach and intestine long enough to be absorbed. The only means of keeping this baby alive was intravenous feeding. He was transferred from the ICN to the general pediatrics ward, with a line into one of his arteries, in the vague hope that, with time, a solution to his fatal problem might be found.

Intravenous feeding was a short-term solution. Eventually, the lines became infected, the arteries collapsed, or fluids infiltrated the surrounding tissue. Ever new sites for the lines had to be found. After a time, none remained close to the body's surface. At that point, a surgeon was called to perform the first in a long series of cut-downs. He repeated the procedure almost weekly for more than two years, always searching deeper for possible sites and thus prolonging the child's life beyond any length of time previously thought possible. But eventually, almost all possible sites for cut-downs were exhausted. All those involved with the infant

195

were extremely uncomfortable with what was taking place. It was then that the ethicist was invited to consult.

The ethicist called attention to the facts, values, and reasoning involved in the case. The facts were plain: medically, nothing could be done to save the child. Medical intervention had merely prolonged his dying. His parents were largely illiterate Hispanics. They did not understand their son's problems, nor the inability of a world-renowned medical center to overcome them. They were continually in touch with their curandero, all of whose potions and herbal remedies were applied to the infant with the full knowledge and encouragement of his physicians, who reasoned that since Western medicine was impotent for this baby, anything the parents wanted to try was acceptable, as long as it was not dangerous.

Three sets of confused and conflicting values were involved in the case: those of the parents, the physicians, and the nurses. The parents were traditional Roman Catholics who believed that life is sacred. The term "quality of life" had little meaning for them. In the surgeon's value system, technical proficiency ranked above ordinary compassion. He concerned himself with performing the incisions as skillfully as possible, without keeping the infant's experience or long-term term prospects in view. But his attitude and behavior assaulted the value system of the nurses, who saw the look of terror in the infant's eyes, had the task of calming him when he became hysterical at the prospect of another cut-down, and cared for him day to day.

The ethicist's task was to clarify the reasoning that had guided treatment so far, and to help arrive at a consensus on what should be done in the future. He noted that, traditionally, several key principles have been honored in medical practice. They include preserving life, alleviating suffering, doing no harm, and allowing the patient as much say as possible in treatment. This baby was too young to speak for himself, and his parents were unaware of the reality of the situation. Occasional efforts had been made to inform them through a translator, but there had been no sustained attempt to bridge the cultural and language gap between them and the hospital staff. It was obvious that preserving life had been ranked above alleviating suffering and doing no harm. But as there was no hope of recovery, it was also obvious that this principle had been inappropriately applied.

The ethicist recommended that "Do no harm" be accepted as the guiding principle in the case, and it was accepted. The boy was transferred to a hospital close to his home, where he was given medication for pain and died soon thereafter.

This ethicist had helped members of the medical team to understand their thinking process better and arrive at a decision that prevented further harm to their patient. That decision, however, came after much harm had already been done, for the boy had been inexorably dying from the day of his birth. Had this issue been confronted in the beginning, much futile suffering would have been averted.[19]

Difficult specific decisions are best made informally, by a small group whose members are well informed, thoughtful, and sensitive to the needs of the patient, the family, and the staff, as well as to the broader value issues. The *Baby Doe* case illustrates the value of consultation and collaboration, preferably among people representing different disciplines and working together. Had this been done when Baby Doe was being treated, the restrictive federal regulations might not have been enacted.

At Stanford, the ethicist takes part in such committees when invited by the caregiving team. In addition, he participates in shaping policy in more formal ways. He is a member of the Medical Center Ethics Committee, formed in 1984, which examines issues with broad ethical implications and makes recommendations. One of this group's achievements was the adoption of a uniform policy on do not resuscitate code orders. It had discovered that sometimes such orders were written without the patient's having been consulted or agreeing. It had also found instances where such orders were called for but were not written; terminally ill patients who were likely to go into cardiac failure were at risk for having their dying artificially prolonged, especially in the cancer unit. The committee drew up a policy designed to prevent both kinds of travesty.

The word *ethics* is often used as a synonym for *morality*, but there is an important distinction between the two. Morality refers to attitudes and actions reflecting a vision of the highest good. That vision may be informed by the Ten Commandments, the person of Jesus, Buddha, Tao, or the U.S. Constitution. Ethics is the discipline that studies and makes proposals about morality. It examines and reflects on moral argument and behavior and seeks for the underpinnings: the quality of evidence brought forward in support of a particular position, the values either implicit or expressed, the kind of reasoning used in arriving at conclusions. Ethics can also suggest what ought to happen in light of the vision of the highest good professed. What attitudes and actions should ideally follow? Why?

Part of the controversy about newborn intensive care grows out of the diversity of moral perspectives brought to bear on it. Ethical analysis can sometimes help to resolve moral conflicts by bringing to light the values and reasoning operating in a given situation.

Those who seek the preservation of fetal and newborn life at all costs generally base their argument on an interpretation of the Bible. They also maintain that to disagree is to deny that life is sacred. But a wide range of views, all based on an interpretation of Scripture and on the principle of life's sacredness, exists among Jewish, Catholic, and Protestant theologians.

In the Jewish community, Orthodox and Conservative rabbis tend to place themselves in the pro-life camp, Reform rabbis in the quality-of-life camp. However, it is difficult to point to any specific statement in explicit support of a particular course or position. Part of the rabbinic tradition is the oral interpretation of what to outsiders may seem unrelated texts and precepts.

Among Catholics, Benedict M. Ashley and Kevin D. O'Rourke enunciate the principle of the sacredness of life when, in support of an absolute opposition to abortion, they state:

> Physicians, nurses, and health care workers should give public witness to their belief in the sanctity of life, the integrity of every person, and the value of human life at every stage of its existence by their compassion and care for their patients.[20]

Among Protestants, Paul Ramsey is perhaps the most articulate and insistent contemporary advocate of an absolute sanctity-of-life view. He stated his position in the preface to his earliest major work on medical ethics, *The Patient as Person* (1970), and has since then repeated it many times in his analysis and writing about particular ethical issues.

> Just as man is a sacredness in the social and particular order, so he is a sacredness in the natural, biological, order. He is a sacredness in bodily life. He is a person who within the ambience of the flesh claims our care. He is an embodied soul or ensouled body. He is therefore a sacredness in the fruits of the generative process. . . . The sanctity of human life prevents ultimate trespass upon him even for the sake of others who are also only a sacredness in their bodily lives.[21]

In 1978 he made plain his stand on the quality-of-life issue: "I'd rather be charged with morally justifying first degree murder . . . than to add a feather's weight on the balance in favor of quality-of-life judgments—unless these are part of a competent patient's balancing determination of goods and harms in his own case.[22] Ramsey excludes the possibility of a similar "balancing determination" in behalf of a newborn.

Thus, supporters of life at all costs can be found in the dominant three faiths in the United States. But all faiths have also produced voices urging that the quality of life to be saved be considered.

Among Christian theologians, Joseph Fletcher, a Protestant, has been outspoken. In a discussion of *euthanasia* (which literally means not "mercy killing" but "allowing someone to have a gracious death"), he has written:

> The traditional ethics based on the sanctity of life—which was the classical doctrine of medical idealism in its prescientific phases—must give way to a code of ethics of the quality of life. This comes about for humane reasons. It is a result of modern medicine's successes, not failures. New occasions teach new duties, time makes ancient good uncouth, as Whittier said. There are many pre-ethical or "metaethical" issues that are often overlooked in ethical discussions. People of equally good reasoning powers and a high respect for the rules of inference still puzzle and even infuriate each other. This is because they fail to see that their moral judgments proceed from significantly different values, ideals, and starting points. If God's will (perhaps "specially revealed" in the Bible or "generally revealed" in [the] Creation) is against any responsible human initiative in the dying process, or if sheer life is believed to be, as such, more desirable than anything else, then those who hold these axioms will not find much merit in any case we might make for either kind of euthanasia—positive or negative. If, on the other hand, the highest good is personal integrity and human well-being, then euthanasia in either form could or might be the right thing to do, depending on the situation.[23]

Theological witnesses can be brought forward to testify on both sides of a debate couched in terms of sanctity versus quality of life. However, there is no intrinsic contradiction between holding life sacred and taking its quality into account. Richard A. McCormick, a Jesuit, has made the point:

> Quality-of-life assessment ought to be made within an overall reverence for life, as an extension of one's respect for the sanctity of

life. However, there are times when preserving the life of one with no capacity for those aspects of life we regard as human, is a violation of the sanctity of life itself.[24]

An absolute and inflexible sanctity-of-life point of view can be a violation of life's sacredness, for it implies that existence alone, without regard for its texture and possible meaningfulness, is absolutely sacred and must always be maintained at all costs. Yet it is clear from the biblical tradition that to regard anyone or anything as an absolute good is to commit idolatry. According to theologian Paul Tillich,

> Idolatry is the elevation of a preliminary concern to ultimacy. Something essentially conditioned is taken as unconditional, something essentially partial is boosted into universality, and something essentially finite is given infinite significance. . . . The conflict between the finite basis of such a concern and its infinite claim leads to a conflict of ultimates; it radically contradicts the biblical commandments. . . .[25]

The biblical tradition has never accorded an absolute value to physical existence. In Christianity, the veneration of martyrs attests to this; they elected to die rather than compromise truth, fidelity to Christ, justice, loyalty to the community, and other values. Their dying has been construed as "witnessing of heroic proportions," which the word *martyr* literally means, and many of them have been beatified as saints.

In the Jewish tradition, Saul's death ("Saul took his own sword and fell upon it"—I Samuel 31:4) contains many of the same elements as Christian martyrdom. Rather than bring dishonor upon his people, Israel, by falling alive into the hands of the Philistines, Saul chose to end his own life. He was later revered for that sacrifice.

The martyrs honored in our secular culture include patriots and prisoners of war who accepted torture and death rather than betray their fellows and their country. They include Barbara Frietschie, immortalized in the poem by John Greenleaf Whittier and memorized by generations of school children. During the Civil War, she leaned out from her window, unfurled the flag, and told Union soldiers:

> "Shoot, if you must, this old gray head
> But spare your country's flag," she said.

She is admired for her defiance, yet she was putting a flag—a piece of cloth—ahead of her own survival.

Philosopher K. Danner Clouser has pointed out that the ambiguity of the sanctity-of-life argument for a life-at-all-costs position allows it to be used against itself: since life *is* so special, it should not be degraded by being forced to continue in degraded form.[26]

Indeed, minimal physical existence alone, without any capacity for mental, emotional, and spiritual awareness, interaction, and development, is a travesty. It mocks, rather than respects, human life in the sacredness of its design and potential fulfillment.

The argument made on the basis of the principle that life is sacred can also be made on the principle "Above all, do no harm." For how is harm to be defined if not by taking into account what are termed quality-of-life considerations? Only by assessing, or attempting to assess, the balance between the positive and negative experiences a child has had, is having, and is likely to have can one decide whether she or he has or has not been harmed—psychically as well as physically—by medical interventions. Such an assessment constitutes a weighing of the quality of the child's life. If such determinations are to be excluded from the moral decision-making process, as the Baby Doe regulations imply, the deontological principle *Primum non nocere* logically must be abandoned. Are those who uphold an absolute sanctity-of-life ethic willing to go this far, to reduce all guiding principles to one—preserving life always and at all costs?

Such are the questions that arise for an ethicist in examining conflicting views of morality as applied to issues in newborn intensive care. The view underlying the Baby Doe regulations rests on a particular moral perspective, one that is alien to much of the population. It also rests on a simple misunderstanding of what happens in the course of intensive care, and what caring means in the ICN environment. To discontinue intensive treatment is not, as the regulations imply, to desist from care. Neither is it, necessarily, to countenance "medical neglect." Caring may assume different forms. At times, intensive care may be appropriate. At other times, care might require what the British call special intervention, that is, everything short of assisted ventilation. At still other times the aim of care could be to provide comfort rather than cure. Albert Jonsen expressed this point more forcibly.

If "do no harm" means having always the motive to care for the other, termination of painful seriously debilitated existence might be considered a "caring act." . . . Due care consists of assessing medical actions in relation to certain goals. It might be argued that sustaining life of low quality is not a goal of medical actions since medicine is concerned only with restoration of health in some functional sense. At this early stage of this difficult discussion, I would suggest that it is legitimate to invoke the "do no harm" maxim as a justification for termination of life.[27]

Richard McCormick, also wrote:

One can and, I believe, should say that the *person* is always an incalculable value, but that at some point continuance in physical life offers the person no benefit. Indeed, to keep "life" going can easily be an assault on the person and his or her dignity.[28]

It is now widely recognized that adults have the right to refuse further medical treatment on quality-of-life grounds.[29] They can seek death with dignity. To deny that same right to newborns is inconsistent. It is also tantamount to surrender to the technological imperative: acceptance of the view that what can be done ought to be done, always, unthinkingly, and without regard for the consequences.

Newborns weighing 500 grams at twenty-four weeks' gestational age can be treated in neonatal intensive care units. But should they be treated aggressively, or given special care, or merely fed, sedated, and kept warm? This question has to be answered with reference to societal needs, priorities, and resources, as well as to the further question, How might the available technology be used in the most humane, compassionate, and ethically responsible way? To move automatically from what can be done to the contention that it ought, therefore, to be done, might in fact violate the sanctity of life, even as it tends to elevate into an absolute the value placed on physical existence alone.

To refuse to consider quality of life in decisions regarding newborns may also mean succumbing to the legal imperative; one powerful force driving physicians to aggressive treatment is the fear that, if they refrain, they will be subject to malpractice suits. Malpractice premiums are becoming prohibitive in some specialities, including obstetrics and gynecology. Until a better way is found to settle differences arising between physicians and patients about appropriate standards of care, defensive medicine will be practiced, and patients will be overtreated and thereby harmed. Fear of being sued is as significant a factor in the inappropriate escalation of high technology interventions as is the technological imperative.

The antithesis of advocates of the sanctity of life, on the one hand, and those who consider quality of life in decision making, on the other, stems in part from confusion over categories. The terms "sanctity of life" and "quality of life" are treated as if they were opposing moral principles. But they are not. They should be regarded as values. The principles with which these values are correlated are, respectively, preserving life and doing no harm. On the basis of the principle of preserving life, life is valued as potentially sacred. (Incidentally, death is valued as potentially sacred as well, for death is part of life, part of what it is to be human, part of our nature and destiny as individuals and as a species.) On the basis of the principle of doing no harm, life of extremely poor quality is valued negatively, since it is injurious to the individual experiencing it. Life of an acceptable quality is valued positively, since it benefits the individual experiencing it. Depending on which principle predominates, the corresponding values will predominate also.

When a diagnosis is certain, treatment options many and effective, and the prognosis hopeful, preserving life might appear to be not only achievable, but also possible without, on balance, inflicting undue harm on the person being treated. When a diagnosis is uncertain, no good treatment options exist, and the prognosis is bleak, trying to preserve life might not only be futile, but might actually damage the individual being treated. In these two opposite cases, "sanctity of life" and "quality of life" play correspondingly divergent roles as values, but are not directly opposed to each other, per se, as the current debate unfortunately tends to suggest.

To resolve the false dichotomy between sacredness and quality-of-life considerations, a broader view is required. The words *quality of life* have become so loaded emotionally, morally, and politically that to use them may well be counterproductive. We need to think of the question in a new way. What is at stake is life's integrity. The issue is respect for life and its integrity. Such respect implies an appreciation of the fact that physical existence alone is, in the end, meaningless and valueless. Its integrity requires a certain richness of texture, a modicum of awareness, interaction with the environment, interpersonal relatedness, autonomy, and the capacity for experiencing joy and pain.

Respect for life and its integrity demands both a recognition of the preciousness of life, which the sanctity-of-life position is concerned to stress, and an emphasis on the importance of life, as distinct from mere existence, insisted on by advocates of a quality-of-life view. Neonatology is a relatively new medical discipline. The instruments for monitoring data for the purpose of making predictions are still crude. As in other fields of rapid technological progress—nuclear power, for instance—some of the consequences of current interventions will not be known for many years. Studies of outcome—particularly long-range outcome—are sparse and, with some categories of babies, nonexistent, because their survival is too recent. But some data does exist. To gather facts, often with the use of public funds, and then to ignore them is not responsible. It is not responsible to say, as C. Everett Koop does in concluding his little book, "I recognize full well the chance for errors in judgment. Because of that I try to err only on the side of life."[30] That disclaimer does not change the consequence; "to err only on the side of life," in context, means to use the tools of medicine to condemn some newborns to a tortured life sentence.

In the history of neonatology, Baby Doe and Baby Jane Doe mark steps in an expanding participation in decision making, and in the search for moral answers to unprecedented questions raised by advances in medical science and technology. A later installment in the continuing story was Baby Fae, for whom the issue was not whether too little was done, but rather the opposite. On October 27, 1984, Dr. Leonard Bailey, a pediatric cardiac surgeon at Loma Linda Hospital in Loma Linda, California, transplanted the heart of a seven-month-old baboon into a two-week-old human infant in a procedure that had never previously been tried.

The baby had been born prematurely, to a twenty-three-year-old single mother, with a fatal defect known as hypoplastic heart syndrome, in which the left side of the heart is underdeveloped and nearly useless. The surgeon had offered the mother what he considered an operation with "therapeutic intent," rather than, as many other medical scientists and practitioners saw it, an experimental procedure with almost no chance of success. The infant died twenty-one days later, as her immune system turned against the implanted heart. A host of ethical questions was again raised; they were debated for days on the front pages of the press and in TV news, and much longer among ethicists and medical practitioners.

What did the parents consent to? Was this an experiment or a therapeutic procedure? If it was an experiment, what was its design? What was it intended to study? What animal research had preceded it? If the treatment was meant as therapeutic, what scientific basis was there for regarding it that way? What results warranted a classification of this procedure as therapy, rather than as research? And further, why did the world learn about Baby Fae only after the fact?

In a situation where the only alternative is death for a child, a request for consent to an experiment said to offer hope may, in itself, be coercive. Aside from this, there is reason to believe, from an examination of the consent form signed by the parents, that the case was presented to them in a biased manner, and that the facts were presented in a veiled form.

The consent document is remarkably deficient in presenting the risks and the unprecedented nature of the proposal the parents were asked to consider. "It is clear from past experience with many such babies [with hypoplastic left heart syndrome] that without surgical help, it is extremely unlikely that your baby will live beyond the first few days or weeks of life," the form stated, implying that surgery can help. However, surgery to correct this condition did not exist. Nor was it the issue here. A cross-species transplant is more than surgery. The form does not inform the parents of this fact, only saying obliquely, "Temporizing operations [unspecified] to extend the lives of babies like yours by a few months have generally been unsuccessful. We believe heart transplantation may offer hope of life for your baby. Laboratory research at Loma Linda University over the past seven years, including over 150 heart transplants in newborn animals, suggests that long-term survival with appropriate growth and development may be possible following heart transplantation during the first week of life."

Nowhere is it stated that the leap from other animals to humans had never been made. We do not even learn, from this consent form, whether such experiments as were conducted in Loma Linda involved crossing species, or how long those animals survived. The enormous danger of Cyclosporine-A, the drug that is used in transplants to avert rejection but has the side effect of damaging the immune system, is not mentioned. Overall, the document pleads a case for the experiment rather than factually presenting the relevant information.

Not all the questions raised by the Baby Fae incident pertain to the treatment of this child and her parents. Some refer to the treatment of the baboon. In recent years, scientific evidence had been accumulating that the differences between humans and simians are far fewer than we had long, and comfortably, believed. We have learned not only that their DNA (genetic coding material) is similar to ours, but also that they seem able to learn to communicate with us through symbol systems we devise. Psychologists have shown that simian babies, like human offspring, fail to thrive when deprived of living contact with others. Filmmakers have caught terror in the eyes of a primate research lab subject when an experimenter approached.

Such information has led to a growing discomfort with the use of primates in research and to a movement for animal rights, which has spread to include scientists as well as laymen. Dr. Bailey was careful to point out to reporters that the baboons in his laboratory were treated with respect, properly anesthetized before their hearts were removed, and kept clean in a well-ventilated space. Yet a feeling of unease, even horror, persisted for some contemplating the issues raised by the Baby Fae story. They asked the question, Is it right to kill other primates so human babies can have their hearts?

Why did this question arise with Baby Fae, when it did not arise during research for coronary artery bypass grafts, heart transplants, and other developments made possible by experiments with animals?

One answer may lie in the fact that the connection had never before been so direct. In none of the previous instances had a heart been lifted out of another animal's body and transplanted directly into a human breast. (Two decades earlier, an attempt was made in South Africa to use chimpanzee hearts in humans, but as aids rather than replacements. That experiment also failed.) In the Baby Fae case, no intermediate step sanitized the issue and obscured the relationship between a human recipient and another primate.

The heart is more than the "biological pump" Dr. Bailey said he had transposed. It is not only more than a pump biologically, it is also an organ surrounded by symbolic and subliminal significance, exemplified by the Sacred Heart of Jesus, the "path with heart" of the Yaqui shaman, the heart of the lion. In our culture, as in others, the heart signifies love, courage, the ability to transcend selfishness. It is through the heart that we connect with others, be they of our own species or another. (Medical anthropologist Margaret Lock of McGill University, who studied Asian and Western medicine in urban Japan, has speculated that such attributions help explain our preoccupation with heart ailments in this country. In Japan, where the Buddhist tradition views the hara [a point below the navel] as a major energy center, the stomach and its malfunctions get comparable attention, she has observed.)

Taking this baboon heart, then, was an act laden with meaning. But Baby Fae's surgeon had not acknowledged its significance. Dr. Bailey explained that baboons are a "lesser form than our own human species," and that they not only were not endangered but in fact were vermin which destroy crops and kill children in their habitat. But since the 1970s, an understanding of ecological interdependence has made a hierarchical view of life obsolete. The reference to vermin evoked memories of justifications offered in earlier times for the killing of Hottentots, slaves, Indians, and others now considered kin.

In light of all this, the issue of whether the Baby Fae operation should have been done might be less important than the spirit in which it was done. Was the baboon heart taken as one cannibalizes a car for its motor? Or was the act done reverently, with due recognition of a life being taken? It seems safe to assume that pain was avoided, as the procedure was medical. But did the surgeon recognize the blood offering of the baboon for the sake of the human baby's possible survival, the advance of medical science, and the surgeons' glory? In other words, was the baboon simply killed, or was it sacrificed?

Native Americans used to thank the buffalo they killed. Bushmen, who paralyze their game with poisoned arrows before killing, first explain that they and their community need the food. In Africa and parts of Asia, medical practice requires offerings of sheep and goats as sacrifices to the spirits. The Aztecs used to rip hearts out of chosen men's breasts for the sake of harmony with the universe and victory in war. In each instance, there was an encounter of being with being and an offering of respect before the kill.

In our society the word *sacrifice* has lost its ceremonial and religious meaning. Though we still speak of young men being sacrificed for their country in battle, the word is more commonly used in price wars: "Sale—sacrifice prices—everything goes." Industrialization, technological process, and the consumer society have obscured, if not obliterated, the terrain of the sacred. But it is being restored to us in a new way by science, which brings fresh evidence of the wondrous connectedness of life, while enabling us to assume unprecedented control over our own reproduction.

The debates about Baby Doe, Baby Jane Doe, and Baby Fae reflect society's confused gropings for a new recognition of the sacred. But the Baby Doe regulations will solve nothing. They are not informed by the realities of decision making in the nursery, nor do they show any cognizance of the limits and possibilities of current medical and biological science. The courts will not lay the debate to rest. "Courts temporal are not ideally suited to resolve problems that originate in the spiritual realm," Justice Irving R. Kaufman of the United States Court of Appeals for the Second Circuit has observed.[31] The subject is sure to remain high on the agenda of the nation's moral concerns.

CHAPTER NINE

The Costs and Benefits

In the few cases here described, the economic costs have been high. When Angela Walker-Shaw was discharged from the Stanford intensive care nursery, her bill was $335,952; her sister's was $158,624. When Matthew Cordell died, his was $530,409. The medical bills for the first eighteen months of Maria de Jesús Rodriguez's life rose above these figures and would continue to mount. Because these infants were born marginally viable, the cost of their care was far in excess of that of the average ICN patient, which was estimated at $12,000 nationwide in one report.[1] But though they do not represent average expenditures per nursery patient, these bills are not rarities. The more premature or sick the baby is at birth, the longer he is likely to be hospitalized, the higher the risk of disabilities, and the steeper the cost of care. In a study conducted at one hospital, 24 percent of infants with the greatest complications represented 60 percent of the total charges.[2]

In 1985, more than $2 billion a year was being spent on newborn intensive care for some 200,000 babies, 6 percent of those born in the United States. But the infant mortality rate had ceased the dramatic decline that had been observed in the 1960s and 1970s and seemed to be stabilizing at about 10.9 deaths per thousand live births, which left the United States further behind Finland (with 6), Japan (6.6), and several other developed nations than it had been thirty years earlier. This country had slipped from seventh place in 1954 to seventeenth by 1982. In 1979, the U.S. Public Health Service had set a goal of nine per thousand for 1990. It seemed unlikely that this goal could be met.

The internationally embarrassing infant mortality rate had been a major reason for launching the development and expansion of intensive care nurseries with federal funds. The subsequent improvement in the statistics seemed to justify the public investment. It should be noted that the improvement occurred at a time when public funds were being spent more liberally than in earlier years for the betterment of health and well-being of poor people, and during the time when legal abortion became more widely available. These and other factors contributed. However, most of the improvement has generally been attributed to the survival of ever smaller infants.

In other countries, where infant mortality rates also declined during this period, major efforts were directed toward maternal health and prevention of prematurity. In Great Britain and Sweden, for example, where medical service is free of charge to patients and resources are allocated by the government, decisions on whether very low-birth-weight infants should be treated aggressively are made on medical grounds alone and infants born weighing less than 750 grams were not routinely treated aggressively.[3]

As technology came upon the biological threshold of fetus at twenty-four to twenty-seven weeks and 500 to 750 grams, the decline of the infant death rate in this country slowed. In addition, an increase in the postneonatal mortality rate (28 days to 12 months), indicated that intensive care had merely postponed death, at great cost, for some infants. Simultaneously, the country walked away from the war on poverty as public attitudes changed and the economy went into a recession.

Low-birth-weight babies account for two-thirds of twenty-three thousand neonatal deaths annually. Yet since the ICNs began and flourished, the incidence of low birth weight had barely changed at all. In 1982, 6.8 percent of all babies and 12.4 percent of black babies in the United States were born weighing less than 2500 grams (5.5 lbs.). In some poor, predominantly black urban areas, almost 30 percent of all births have been reported as premature. Though there are ethnic and racial variations in prematurity rates—Asians and American Indians have low rates, blacks have higher ones than Hispanics and whites—the clearest links are with low educational status, poverty, and lack of prenatal care: poor women who lack schooling and adequate prenatal care are most likely to have premature infants.

In its 1985 report, the Institute of Medicine Committee to Study the Prevention of Low Birthweight estimated that provision of adequate care to the 3 million women aged fifteen to thirty-nine on public assistance in 1980 could have reduced their rate of premature delivery from 11.5 percent to 9 percent and saved at least $28.6 million in public funds, or $3.38 for each additional $1.00 spent on prenatal care. At the time, the committee estimated, the medical costs of the 12,719 infants born to these women required more than $188.23 million in the first year alone, exclusive of the costs of institutionalizing severely disabled survivors. By spending $12.1 million, we could have achieved a total saving of $40.91 million, the committee stated. The total costs of prenatal care for one woman were estimated to be $500 to $800, less than half the daily cost of intensive care. The committee recommended a program including improved access to prenatal care, expanded prenatal services, better preparation for pregnancy through health education, family-planning services, birth control information for teenagers, and identification of women at high risk.

In May 1985, a ten-member group appointed by the National Institutes of Health noted that prematurity and low birth weight continue to be correlated with an increased risk of both cerebral palsy and mental retardation. It suggested that the bulk of resources in this field be directed toward preventing low birth weight, premature delivery, and asphyxia.

Such reports did not break new ground; they merely added documentation to what had long been known: prevention is more effective than rescue after the fact. Yet ICNs continued to proliferate and expand, as did other areas of medical technology, while the simpler, more humane, and much more effective approach of prevention continued to be neglected. The reasons for this discrepancy lay partly in the American character, partly in the fact that hospitals, medical researchers, and others had an interest in the prevailing course.

Americans have a strong bias in favor of high-technology medical crisis interventions, preferring to invest in these at the expense of possible low-key efforts to maintain health or alleviate chronic problems. This is evident in, for example, the enormous expenditures on heart transplants and artificial hearts as compared to the resources expended in improving diet and habits associated with heart disease. It is evident in the fact that $2 billion a year has been spent on kidney dialysis and kidney transplants for sixty-five thousand patients, and $125 million on five hundred liver transplants, while an estimated 4 million children had inadequate access to basic medical care. The $114,000 average cost of a heart transplant could, by one estimate, pay for health screenings for six thousand children.[4]

The public preference is the background against which contemporary medicine has evolved. In the field of neonatology, timing was also a factor in catalyzing growth. When the new medical specialty came into being, public funding was freely available for research and development in science and medicine, so the high costs of intensive care could be applied directly to research protocols rather than having parents, third-party payers, or the wider community pay directly. Had neonatology come onto the medical stage fifteen years later, in the early 1980s rather than the late 1960s, different economic constraints might well have inhibited its progress and mitigated against its proliferation.

Economic factors continue to generate momentum for expansion. For medical researchers, the ICN continues to be a "highly prized research lab," according to psychiatrist Eugene Brody. It provides a captive population and a contained environment that allows for the structure of plans with controllable variables, in comparison, for example, with studies of infant development beyond the ICN, where data-gathering procedures are far more complex. (Research on infant development is neglected within the nursery as well: funds are more readily available for research on pharmaceutical and technological interventions. Stanford did not have a developmentalist on its neonatology staff in 1985.)

For hospitals, the ICN constitutes one of the more lucrative sources of income. In recent years, as competition among hospitals has grown, many have rushed to set up intensive care units in a bid for this revenue. The rush has also been fueled by a surplus of neonatologists: one-third of all pediatricians who seek postdoctoral training choose neonatology, according to Dr. Philip Sunshine. The announcement of a staff opening usually brings flurries of applications.

The proportion of revenue earned for a hospital through neonatology is consistently higher than the proportion of licensed beds devoted to newborn intensive care. At the Stanford University Medical Center, in 1984, the cost per day for an ICN bed was $1550. The hospital had 663 licensed beds, twenty-five of which, or 3.7 percent, were designated for newborn intensive care. In fiscal 1982–1983, revenues from the ICN were $9.47 million, 4.4 percent of a total $217.57 million in hospital revenues. In fiscal 1983–1984, the amount rose to $11.09 million, or 4.7 percent of total revenues of $236.44 million.

The per-bed cost is only part of the income generated through intensive care. Above that, there are charges for laboratory tests, CT scans, ultrasound, other procedures and services. For an infant receiving the most aggressive care, the daily charge in 1985 was over $2400 at Stanford. Most high-risk infants begin their nursery stay in this category of care, and some stay in it for prolonged periods.

In addition, 82 percent of the faculty-generated income for patient care in pediatrics has come through the ICN and is shared by the entire department, according to a senior neonatologist. Some of the neonatologists' budget requests go unmet, however. Significant among these have been the request for a developmentalist and for more social service staff time.

Of about six hundred intensive care nurseries nationwide, 30 to 40 percent are associated with research units in university medical centers. Either through research grants they help generate or revenue accruing directly to the hospitals, these beds are highly effective income producers. There is no national data, however, on the utilization of newborn intensive care. All estimates are based on limited figures. According to an estimate by Victor R. Fuchs and Leslie Perreault, normal newborn care for 3,496,000 infants in 1982 totaled $1.5 billion, including hospital and physician costs, while the expenditures for 185,000 infants in intensive care were $2.2 billion. Total expenditures for children in the first year of life were estimated at $6.5 billion. Sixty percent of the total went to newborn care.[5] Marginally viable infants have many medical needs after the newborn nursery and usually require rehospitalization during the first year. Only 10 percent of the total spent nationally on health care for children in the first year of life went to well-baby care, preventive care, and medical care for problems not requiring hospitalization.

Neonatal intensive care is big business. In a time when even not-for-profit hospitals face severe economic constraints due to declining numbers of patients, fewer patient-days per annum, and fixed reimbursement systems of billing, the economic advantages of providing high-technology intensive care for neonates outweigh any commitment to preventing prematurity and the incidence of very low-birth-weight infants—however cost-effective that may be for society as a whole. From the hospital's point of view, the two issues are not even in the same ballpark. The interests of hospitals and those of society appear to be directly in conflict at this point. Hospitals depend for most of their revenue on sophisticated services such as neonatal, cardiac, and medical/surgical intensive care; society's need to conserve shrinking resources could best be served by preventive medicine.

A few cost-benefit analyses have been published, suggesting that intensive care for infants in the very low-birth-weight category is not only medically and ethically questionable because of the high risk of disabilities among survivors, but also that it is economically unsound from a societal perspective.

In a Canadian study, published in the *New England Journal of Medicine* in June 1983, Michael H. Boyle and others at McMaster University Medical Center, Hamilton, Ontario, evaluated the economic aspects of neonatal intensive care of infants weighing 1000 to 1499 grams before and after the introduction of a regional neonatal intensive care program in Hamilton-Wentworth County, an urban, industrial county in southern Ontario, which had a birth and infant mortality rate typical for the United States, Canada, and England. They found that the greatest increase in survival rate, the greatest societal costs, and the highest morbidity occurred in the lowest birth-weight groups. Intensive care for babies weighing less than 1000 grams represented a net drain on society's resources, consuming more than it created.[6] The study was based on infants in ICNs between 1973 and 1977. Improvements in treatment would no doubt have shown a higher threshold later. But since that time, smaller babies have been surviving, adding to societal costs. In addition, an increase in postneonatal deaths was reported. If included in the above cost-benefit studies, the data would have added to the cost per survivor.

In a later study in Rhode Island, reported in *Pediatrics* in July 1984, Dr. Donna-Jean B. Walker amd her colleagues estimated the total costs of medical care required by infants of very low birth weight admitted to Women and Infants Hospital of Rhode Island between January 1977 and December 1981. They found that the total costs per survivor with a birth weight between 600 and 699 grams was $362,992, in hospital, physician, and long-term care expenses. For those weighing 700 to 799 grams, it was $116,221. The costs dropped with rising birth weight: babies of 800 to 899 grams cost $101,356; those between 900 and 999 required $40,647.

The authors noted that infants weighing more than 900 grams had a greater than 50 percent chance of survival and an 85 percent chance of developing normally and that their estimated average lifetime earnings, per survivor, exceeded the costs of their medical care. Infants weighing less than 900 grams, however, had high mortality and morbidity rates, and were not likely to earn as much in their lifetimes as their medical care would cost.[7]

No study is available on costs and benefits in terms of intangible, noneconomic factors, such as the effect on families of the death of children after a few months of survival,[8] the impact of disability on parents and siblings, and the gains in medical knowledge. However, the economic measures point the way toward gauging some of these.

Adequate follow-up of ICN graduates is scarce. The report *Preventing Low Birthweight* points out: "According to the NCHS [National Center for Health Statistics] and the Centers for Disease Control (CDC), no national data system is currently being planned to look systematically at the relationship between low birthweight and subsequent morbidity." This is a glaring omission, grounds for an argument that ICN technology is being applied as an uncontrolled experiment, without assumption of responsibility for its consequences.

It is not irrelevant that only a tiny fraction of the total neonatal intensive care costs are borne by parents of the infant patients. According to a financial officer at the Stanford University Medical Center, up to 95 percent of all charges are met by insurance companies, by MediCal, the federal-state program for indigents, by Medicare, the federal program for the disabled and the elderly, by California Children's Services, a state program serving disabled children, and by various charitable organizations. The amount privately paid consists almost exclusively of deductibles. This means that society pays both directly and indirectly.

However, the picture changes after the child has been discharged from the ICN. Resources for the medical and other needs of frail or disabled ICN graduates are far more scarce than resources to keep them alive at birth. A substantial number of infants born at the border of viability have permanent deficits, deficiencies, and disabilities, physical or mental or both. In a study originated at Stanford and published in *Pediatrics* in May 1982, the authors reported that "for infants with birth weights below 750 gm, the prognosis remains poor." For infants with birth weights in the 751 to 1000 gram range who were born between 1977 and 1980 and cared for in a neonatal intensive care center, the survival rate was 72 percent; the probability of significant handicaps among survivors was estimated at 30 percent. Ten percent of these infants, especially those requiring ventilator support, were not expected to grow into self-sufficiency.[9]

The following year, the authors reported that three of the eighty-four infants in the original study had died later during long hospitalization and five had died after discharge (one with chronic lung disease, two with pneumonia, one with sudden infant death syndrome [SIDS] and one with congenital heart disease.) Four did not participate in the follow-up. Of the remaining seventy-two, four had severe and fourteen moderate handicaps. Of the eighteen infants in the study born with a birth weight less than 600 grams, seventeen died (fourteen within the first day), and the one survivor was developmentally delayed.[10]

Other research has produced similar results. Toshiko Hirata reported, in the May 1983 issue of *Pediatrics,* that 50 percent of infants born weighing between 501 and 750 grams could be expected to live. Of these, 11 percent were expected to be retarded or have neurologic problems, 11 percent would have physical handicaps that render them nonfunctional, and 33 percent would not be normal.[11]

Infants of very low birth weight, 1500 grams or less, constitute 1.15 percent of all births. Their survival requires the greatest expenditures, with the cost increasing with their decreasing size. They are twenty times more likely than normal-weight children to die after the first month of life, and account for up to 30 percent of deaths during this period. They remain three times as likely as those of normal weight to have neurological disabilities, including cerebral palsy, according to a report by Dr. Marie C. McCormick in the January 10, 1985, *New England Journal of Medicine.* "Less well established is the risk of other developmental problems, especially those related to success in school," she writes. "It does appear, however, that low birth weight is a predictor of school failure, and this may be particularly true for infants who are small for their gestational age." A key factor may be asphyxia at birth, rather than the birth weight itself, she adds.[12]

The effect of the survival of high-risk infants on their families has received little attention from researchers. Dr. McCormick points out that such studies as have been published give cause for concern. She cites one study, which found high levels of behavioral problems among preschool children who were of very low weight at birth, and also found that these problems were associated with decreased performance on standardized IQ tests. The author of this report, Sibylle K. Escalona of the Rose F. Kennedy Center for Research in Mental Retardation and Human Development, Albert Einstein College of Medicine, Yeshiva University, New York, also reported that "socioeconomic status exerts an overwhelming influence upon the later cognitive development of children." Infants who are at risk biologically are more susceptible to adverse environmental influences.[13]

It is highly relevant, therefore, to consider what services are offered to families, children, and particularly to the disabled and to their families in the society that is creating this new population with special problems and needs.

In 1985, disabled infants and children were living in hospitals throughout the country because they had no place to go, either because their parents could not get the assistance required to keep them at home or because no residential placement was available. One such child was Kareem Loatman, who had spent all but six months of his four and a half years at Boston City Hospital and was still dependent on a respirator and a tracheostomy. He had been sent home twenty-one days after birth but was rehospitalized at seven months with a fever, which was followed by a collapsed lung and continuing respiratory difficulties. From a medical point of view, his doctor said, he could have been discharged three years previously, if special home care were provided. But the financial and logistical obstacles could not be overcome. The *Boston Globe* reported about Kareem on February 28, 1985, calling him "technology's child."

In some states, pediatric units have been established in geriatric nursing homes to accommodate children with multiple severe handicaps, including those from the new population of marginal newborns who grow up as technology's children.[14] Massachusetts first licensed four such units in 1971, to provide skilled and intermediate nursing care to 421 children, after parents of children living in large wards of state institutions filed a class action suit arguing that the care provided violated a constitutionally guaranteed "right to treatment" for institutionalized persons. The suit prompted the Massachusetts Department of Mental Health to close admissions to the state institutions for children under six. A report on patients in nursing homes in 1983 found that "low standards of care and financial disincentives have resulted in less than optimal educational and rehabilitative services."[15]

How newborn intensive care has affected the incidence of disability in the general population remains unclear. Several researchers have reported observing an upward trend in handicapping conditions among children, but the explanations for this have remained elusive. According to the National Health Interview Survey, conducted for the National Center for Health Statistics, the proportion of children with limitations of activity as a result of chronic illness nearly doubled between 1960 and 1980. Two million children suffered some degree of limitation of their activities because of health or disability in 1981, according to the survey, compared to one million between 1958 and 1961. However, this perceived increase does not necessarily reflect any actual increase. It may be explainable as the consequence of changes in the data-gathering process and by other factors, including the greater availability of special education classes and greater national attention to learning disabilities. Studies by Paul W. Newacheck, Peter P. Budetti, and others looked at the National Survey data and found that much of the change could be attributed to the manner in which the survey was conducted.[16] In a 1981 Office of Technology Assessment report on costs and effectiveness of neonatal intensive care, Budetti pointed out that "morbidity data are not collected on a routine basis in the United States. Thus, the incidence of problems and trends over time in the general population cannot be determined." Such studies of ICN survivors as exist are mostly based on data from individual nurseries and are often not comparable.[17]

From such data as can be found, it appears that the net effect of newborn intensive care so far has been to leave the incidence of disability in the general population basically unchanged. Many children who would have survived with disabilities before the ICNs now emerge intact, but a new population of disabled children has been created from the "rescue" of very small or sick infants. Staff at the California Children's Services facilities have observed that, among their clients, children with multiple handicaps have been growing in number. The Baby Doe regulations are contributing toward the increased survival of extremely disabled children.

What is particularly disturbing to some development specialists is the apparently high number of neurological and sensory deficits among babies who are born on the threshold of viability. However, data on the incidence of learning, language, and behavior disorders is far less reliable than data on blindness, for instance. Disabilities that involve higher neurological functions are often not discovered in infancy but can turn up years later, especially when the child enters school. In studies, such handicaps tend to be classified as moderate or minor, though they are likely to affect the ability to communicate and to learn.

Among the nation's disabled, ICN graduates are a significant recent, though tiny, subgroup. In 1984, four federal programs— Supplemental Security Income (SSI), Social Security Disability Insurance, Medicare, and Medicaid—cost more than $32 billion in outlays to people with disabilities. Infants become eligible for SSI at age one.

Though expenditures fail to meet needs, in the 1980s they were being cut back both on the national and state levels. In 1981 President Ronald Reagan ordered his staff to trim the federal budget for special education by 30 percent and was prevented from so doing by a slim margin in Congress. That same year, five hundred thousand disabled people receiving federal payments were struck from the rolls. About 60 percent succeeded in having their benefits restored after appeal, but they did not receive any support during the legal process. Medicaid has been cut back in nearly every state. Community health centers suffered federal fund cuts averaging 30 to 45 percent in 1982. As a result, 28 percent of the centers (239) either limited services or closed.[18]

The resources assigned to take care of the disabled population are shrinking. The Reagan administration has steadily pursued a policy of decreasing federal spending on social services, urging the states and voluntary organizations to provide what is lacking. However, the gap created by the withdrawal of federal funding has not been filled. This is true not just of funds for the disabled, but also in the broad spectrum of health care and in programs affecting children. Between 1979 and 1982, the number of poor children rose more than 30 percent, from 10 million to 13.3 million, according to a census bureau study.

Children constitute 40 percent of the poor in the United States, according to government data. Federal spending reductions between 1981 and 1984 have, in general, affected children, young people, and families while sparing the elderly. The economic status of the elderly is rising while that of children has fallen. Senator Daniel Patrick Moynihan of New York has observed that "the U.S. today may be the first society in history where children are much worse off than adults."[19]

The deteriorating health status of children and of childbearing women, particularly in areas of high unemployment, has been observed by a growing number of researchers. There are reports of a large increase in anemia in pregnant women and in the number and percentage of women who receive no prenatal care, or none before the third trimester. Medicaid in 1985 covered only 52 percent of the poor, as compared with 65 percent in 1976. Thirty-five million people—10 million more than in 1977, were without health insurance in 1985.[20]

This is the context in which the expenditure of more than $2 billion annually on saving frail children through intensive care has to be considered. It should be weighed in relation to resources allotted to support all persons in the society who are unable to maintain their well-being autonomously. These include the disabled, the poor, the retarded, the mentally ill, the aged. As programs for all society's dependents are increasingly judged in terms of cost-effectiveness, it is ever more clear that preventing preterm births is a more rewarding approach—in terms of dollars as well as saving lives and helping children grow up healthy—than is neonatal intensive care for very low-birth-weight infants.

How much is being spent for this purpose nationally is not known. No study exists, which is further evidence of neglect of interest in the area. Dr. Arthur Salisbury, vice president for medical services of the March of Dimes Birth Defects Foundation, ventured an estimate: about $5 million nationwide—less than 0.4 percent of the outlay for neonatal intensive care. In light of the cost-effectiveness estimates proffered by the Committee to Study the Prevention of Low Birthweight, this represents reckless disregard for economic common sense.

Among experimental programs that have achieved a reduction in preterm births is one funded by a $1 million grant from the March of Dimes and directed by Dr. Robert K. Creasy. Begun in 1978 at the University of California at San Francisco and since expanded to five major cities, it focuses on teaching women to identify early signs of labor, then treating them with tocolytic (obstetric) drugs to stop labor. Preliminary results showed that during the first two years, the number of women who recognized the early signs increased more than fourfold. A significant reduction in preterm deliveries was observed. Dr. Salisbury said that this study will probably catalyze others, but that those interested in the model are waiting for the final results, expected in 1987.

It appears that the standard of proof of effectiveness being applied for programs designed to prevent prematurity is much more rigorous than it is for the use of various aggressive interventions with newborns in the nursery. Many of the therapies used routinely in ICNs have been little studied and their long-term consequences are unknown.

Prenatal care is provided routinely and without charge in some advanced nations that have a better record on infant survival. In France, where reduction in the prematurity rate has been a national goal since 1971, the government reported an overall drop in preterm births from 8.2 percent in 1973 to 5.3 percent in 1982.[21] A diverse and experimental approach has been used to achieve the goal. One tactic has been the use of cash payments as incentives to women to participate in prenatal care programs. Employers are required to provide leave to women whose physicians order them to stop working during pregnancy. The employee either receives full salary or an equivalent public subsidy.

Such policies are in sharp contrast with practices in the United States, which is an exception among industrialized countries in not having a law to provide basic health services and social support to working women during childbearing, noted Dr. C. Arden Miller, chairman of maternal and child health, School of Public Health, University of North Carolina at Chapel Hill. "Indeed, the policy in the U.S. is to treat pregnancy and childbearing as if they were disabilities," Dr. Miller wrote in the July 1985 issue of *Scientific American*. "Benefits are provided to such women in the same way and to the same limited extent as they are for illnesses. Even that assurance has prevailed only since 1978, when Congress spelled it out in the Pregnancy Discrimination Act."

In Finland, a woman is entitled to eleven months of paid maternity leave. In Sweden, she gets a year, which can begin before the birth. Extensive birth control information is provided to teenagers so that "we don't have a problem of unwed teen mothers" (a major correlating factor in prematurity), according to Dr. Niels C. R. Raïha, chairman of the department of pediatrics at the University of Lund, Malmö, Sweden. High-quality medical care is free and "so well organized that even the high income mothers go to the prenatal clincs." The rate of infant mortality and of prematurity are half the U.S. rate. The rate of teenage pregnancy and teenage abortion is low, though the overall rate of abortion is high. The rate of very low-birth-weight infants is half that of the United States. While the point is often made that the United States has a much more ethnically diverse population, Dr. Raïha said that southern European and Turkish guest workers and immigrants have rates as good as those of native Swedes.

Dr. Miller writes that the Public Health Service goal of a nine per thousand infant death rate could be met by 1990. "The means . . . are not mysterious, but they require the implementation of certain public policies that are not even being seriously considered." These include "assured access to comprehensive perinatal care, guaranteed maternity leaves for all working pregnant women and recent mothers, job protection during the leave and cash benefits equal to a significant portion of wages during the leave. These measures can be promoted on the basis of humanitarian concern, social equity, cost-effectiveness and even national security to the extent that it will depend on a coming generation both vigorous and productive."[22]

At present, the women who get the best prenatal care in the United States are those at the lowest risk of losing an infant.

When the investment of extraordinary resources in intensive care for marginal newborns is matched by extraordinary support later, it can sometimes bring much fulfillment to parents. Some families can afford what the task requires physically, psychically, and financially. The parents of Angela Walker-Shaw managed. Whether the Cordells could have is questionable, for their circumstances were more constrained. The advances in fertility obstetrics and neonatology have created new options. But these options are, by and large, luxuries.

Among well-to-do couples who are willing to go to great lengths to conceive and bear children were Laura and Jim Petras, successful entrepreneurs in their mid-thirties who found happiness in the birth of a daughter at twenty-four weeks' gestation—the very earliest that a fetus/baby can be kept alive outside the womb. Laura had had several miscarriages before Veronica was born, weighing 650 grams (1 lb. 7 oz.). The parents' private doctor supported their demand that the ICN physicians go further than they thought was wise in treating the baby, and Veronica surprised everyone by surviving and going home with oxygen support.

The Petras's home is spacious and secluded, atop a forested mountain overlooking the ocean. There, with professional pediatric nursing care—around the clock at first, then less often—Veronica continued to improve and grow. At one year she was off the oxygen, the nurses had been replaced by a housekeeper, she was doing well cognitively, and she was beginning to crawl. Though too little is known about babies born so early to predict long-term outcome, at one year the outlook was good. And certainly the parents were providing every opportunity for her healthy development, using their considerable skills and resources. Laura devoted herself to the baby's well-being as completely as she had earlier to the business she and her husband had founded and built into a prosperous concern. Their health insurance policy, which covered all the medical expenses, had no lifetime ceiling. Despite another miscarriage after Veronica's birth, Laura was hoping for yet another child. When asked if she had considered adoption, she said she had not, explaining, "I guess the best way to put it is . . . We want a baby of our own."

Another lucky family who desperately wanted a baby of their own were the Harans, Bryan and Amy, a middle-class couple in their late thirties. Their problem was infertility. A few years earlier, nothing could have helped them conceive. But in 1983, microsurgery on Amy's fallopian tubes was followed, only three months later, by pregnancy. Bryan Jr. arrived at twenty-six weeks, weighing 880 grams (1 lb. 15 oz.). During his five-month ICN tenure, Amy spent many hours daily at his side. She and her husband made special efforts to become known and liked among the nurses, to guarantee that their baby received the utmost attention. That came easily, for they were friendly and grateful for what was being done.

The plan all along had been that Amy would be a full-time homemaker if there were children. She took on that role joyfully, assisted in the baby's care for several months by professional nurses. Bryan Jr. became the central figure in the home. Guests were kept to a minimum for more than a year and nobody with a sign of a cold came near the baby, not even a parent. As Bryan approached his second birthday, he was still on oxygen nights but was a friendly, active child. Amy was again pregnant—and past the gestational age at which Bryan had born. She and her husband had been willing to risk another premature birth for the sake of having a larger family.

For this family, the baby was a great blessing. His birth brought the parents closer together and inspired the father to peak performance in his work. At the end of the first year of his son's life, Bryan Sr. had broken a sales record for his company and been named employee of the year. The group insurance policy covered all expenses, including the home nursing. But at the end of that same year, the insurance carrier refused to renew the employee group contract with the firm unless payments were doubled. Bryan Jr. was one of the causes.

Both Veronica Petras and Bryan Haran, Jr., are receiving the care necessary for achieving their full potential. Research by Sarale E. Cohen and Arthur H. Parmelee has shown that social factors were the most significant among several variables affecting how premature children grow. They are more important than birth weight, length of gestation, or length of hospitalization after birth.

Most people love their children and try to give them the best possible circumstances for growth. But not everyone has the resources required by such fragile beings, especially when deficits in the family cause a baby to be born threshold-viable.

Very different from the Petras and Haran histories is that of Harry Mann, born seriously asphyxiated, with a brain bleed. He was diagnosed as suffering from fetal alcohol syndrome and later as a failure to thrive.

Under California law, a child growing up in a home where the principal caretaker is an alcoholic is considered an abused child. When the mother's sickness came to light through Harry's birth, the father, Shawn, faced the choice of losing custody of the baby, and his two-year-old daughter, or leaving his wife. He chose the children and moved into his mother's modest apartment. His salary, $1300 a month, compelled economy.

For Shawn, this damaged, very premature boy's survival meant dropping out of night school and building his entire life around the care of an infant. He and his mother both worked in a stockroom at a large corporation. His mother changed to the night shift so she could care for the children while Shawn was at work. They devised a tight schedule. Every weekday morning, at 6:30 A.M., Shawn's mother drove her son to work, taking the children along. On her way back, she dropped the girl at day care. Then she drove home with the baby and usually caught some sleep while Harry napped. Before 3:00 P.M., she packed the baby into the car again to pick up her son when he got off. He would take the car, collect his daughter, and go home to be with the children until it was time to get his mother again, at 11:00 P.M.

Many families of limited means organize their lives in similar fashion while their children are small. The difference here was that Harry was not about to become a normal child on his way to nursery school. At one year, he weighed only 9.5 pounds and still seemed to Shawn like a newborn. He could not sit up, did not talk. He was deaf and at risk for cerebral palsy. His mental potential was a big question mark. There was a strong possibility that he would be a dependent for the rest of his life.

Besides this big worry, there was also the fact that Shawn's health insurance did not cover all of Harry's considerable expenses and required that he select physicians from a panel that did not include the doctors who had seen Harry at Stanford. When the baby was one year old, Shawn had a stack of doctors' bills totaling over $9000, plus others he did not want to total because they were so far beyond his means.

Will Shawn and his mother continue indefinitely to sacrifice most of their other interests and activities for the sake of this baby? Should they? Will they have the strength and endurance? Was there a missed opportunity earlier in the story of this baby where the damage might have been prevented, at lesser cost and greater benefit for all concerned?

A common factor in the sagas of many infants who come through the ICN is lack of adequate care for the mother during pregnancy. A case in point is Sandy Nelson, who gave birth to twin boys, each under two pounds, after bearing two normal and healthy sons. She was twenty-seven and in good health, but her pregnancy was a time of extreme demands on her energy. In addition to taking care of her family and a dying relative, she worked full time at a job that required her to stand all day and lift heavy objects. When she started to bleed and went to a doctor, he told her to stay in bed for two days, then return to work. Another doctor might have advised bed rest. Another woman, with fewer pressures bearing down on her, might have taken the rest without being told.

One twin died, and the other, Joel, survived, developmentally delayed. Two years later, the family was struggling to survive on one paycheck, instead of the two that had just sufficed before the baby arrived. Sandy took in another child for day care after school. It was one of the ways she managed, along with learning new recipes for beans and finding cheap ways to spend time with the boys on weekends when, three days from payday, she was left with only a five-dollar bill. Dove hunting was good, and also fishing. They had the advantage of bringing in dinner sometimes. The gas to get there could go on credit.

She would rather have had a job; she was too energetic to stay in the little trailer home at the edge of town all day, but there really was no other option. Part-time jobs were scarce in her town, she had no car when Bruce was at work, and Joel needed her. He might continue to need her. During follow-up visits to Stanford, she had been urged to enroll him in infant stimulation classes for the developmentally delayed. But, although she worries about him, she is convinced that he is growing fine, at his own pace. It is possible to see her attitude as positive thinking or as denial. She is a loving, optimistic mother. She and her family are also, more than they were earlier, under stress. Was there a point in her pregnancy when it could have been helped to reach term?

For most families, taking care of infants with many special needs is a hardship, even when the outcome, by medical standards, is good. The whole family may need to shoulder many financial and other demands that come with such a baby. Even when services are available in the community, and the family manages to get to them, the presence of a child requiring extraordinary care may be a burden too heavy for some to manage if they are already under stress in other ways, especially economically. This fact helps to explain why premature and damaged infants are more likely than others to be abused children.

Neonatal intensive care for borderline babies may well be a luxury that many families cannot afford, even if a third party pays all the medical bills. But once a baby is rescued and home in the parents' arms, that issue becomes academic. At the moment of birth, many parents, including Sandy Nelson, were prepared to see their fetus/babies die. They knew they were too early. Some thought they were having a miscarriage. But deliberate efforts were made by the hospital staff to bond the mothers to these unready beings. Afterward, there was no choice for the parents but to do all they could, no matter what the personal cost. Sometimes, that cost may be not only economically but also humanly excessive.

It has been observed that this country is moving toward a two-tiered system of medical care, in which enormously expensive and sophisticated technology will be available to some while basic services shrink for others. In August 1985, ABC-TV's "Nightline" featured a story about a nineteen-year-old woman who was found to be an excellent candidate for a heart transplant at Stanford University. She and her parents were told that, without a transplant, she had only about three months to live. The transplant could be performed, but the parents first had to put up $125,000. The parents mortgaged the small restaurant they owned but were unable to raise the money. The young woman died on the ninety-first day—precisely on the three-month deadline foreseen by Stanford physicians. Meanwhile, middle-aged people who could raise the money were fitted with recycled hearts.

On November 30, 1984, the *San Jose Mercury News* carried an Associated Press story from Fort Worth, Texas, reporting that a doctor who delivered premature twin girls to a couple with no medical insurance had to call seven hospitals before one agreed to take them, but only after the hospital in which they were born guaranteed the bill.

While those lucky enough to be affluent or well insured can extend their lives through avant-garde medicine, basic medical care is being denied to many others. Yet medical costs and insurance premiums are rising as the population at large is asked to absorb special costs for a few.

This kind of inequality is likely to continue and become ever more aggravated unless steps are taken to adjust the balance that is now weighted so much more on the side of high-technology interventions, including newborn intensive care, than toward routine, normal, humane health care, equitably distributed.

CHAPTER TEN

What of Those

We Force to Live?

What happens to infants who are "salvaged" in the intensive care nurseries only to grow up as permanent dependents? That question is growing in urgency as more infants who would have died at birth without heroic medical efforts are sent out into communities to grow up disabled. Those who make decisions on their behalf at birth have to consider what resources are available for these infants further along in life, and what happens to their families. We cannot demand aggressive life-saving treatment for borderline babies without also demanding that these children receive the support they require to live as well as possible.

Yet there is a notable imbalance between the resources invested in the initial "rescue" and the follow-through, just as there is a growing imbalance between "rescue" and prevention of prematurity. Services for the disabled have been cut back nationally, even as the need for them has risen. To examine only the actions in the intensive care nursery when discussing the issues concerning borderline-viable babies would be to indulge in an exercise in tunnel vision—the kind of vision that creates many of the problems here reviewed.

Few ICN physicians ever visit the facilities to which their tragic newborn survivors are eventually sent. They should, but their charge is to work professionally within the nursery. We cannot also expect them to become the concerned caretakers of the children they save. We as a society, however, we who set policy both directly and indirectly through our ballots, must consider the larger picture. In an effort to learn how the more seriously damaged infants live, we look at the George Miller Junior Memorial

Center in Concord, California, a day school that some of the Stanford ICN alumni attend.

Everything about Cathy Adachi is kinetic. She talks not only with words—though her gift for language is considerable—but with her whole body. Emotion moves in lights and shadows across her face, her arms fly outward or toward you, bursts of energy flash through her small, finely articulated hands and out through the tips of her long fingers. She is a natural mime, so even if you did not know the language, you'd get the drift of her meaning.

When she laughs, she holds nothing back. She loves to laugh. Unlike many people whose laughter is buried deep and only comes up, choked and struggling, when they really can't help themselves (or in the movies, where it's dark and private), Cathy Adachi's laughter is right there, ready to burst anytime, lighting up her face, causing her to toss her long shining black hair.

Because Adachi expresses herself so freely with her body, it seems both odd and fitting that she should be working with children who are almost totally denied such expression. At the George Miller Junior Memorial Center, where Adachi is a physical therapist, children cannot move without assistance, or, if they can, their movements are spastic, random sequences of bizarre posturing or radically inappropriate for their chronological age. These children are developmentally disabled to such an extreme degree that most cannot perform the simplest self-care functions, and probably never will. They can continue to attend public school here, free of charge, until their twenty-second birthday, at which point they may be transferred to an adult program if one is accessible to them. They will be dependents their entire lives, and most, if not all, will eventually live in publicly funded foster homes or institutions.

Most of the children who are bused in, five days a week, from Contra Costa County communities, were born disabled, though some are victims of later illness or accidents. Some had genetic defects that were apparent from the beginning; some seemed normal at birth, their problems not having been diagnosed until much later, even as late as age five. Some were traumatized during gestation or birth and survived because of heroic measures taken in intensive care nurseries. These children now attend George Miller and similar schools, whether they live at home, in foster care, or in pediatric nursing homes.

Adachi and the rest of the George Miller staff do not spend much time researching the elaborate details of children's histories, which are not relevant to treatment in their current circumstances. The staff's job is to coax along such potential as the children may have, to help them toward as much autonomy and enjoyment as possible—even if it involves only the ability to bring a spoon to the mouth or to crawl toward a desired object.

The children Adachi works with are those for whom a physician has prescribed physical therapy. The state regulations that make physical therapy available through California Children's Services stipulate that the recipients must demonstrate improvement. But by ages seven to nine, the progress of most of these children begins to decelerate sharply. They have developed functionally as far as they are able. The provision of physical therapy may prevent scoliosis, painful contractures, and hip dislocation. But this service is often classified as maintenance rather than progress. The older the children, the less direct therapy service they are likely to receive.

The George Miller school is a pleasant single-story complex, with large windows opening on greenery, situated in one of the more prosperous suburban communities east of San Francisco. Among the best of its type, it was designed to be a collaborative venture between the county hospital and the school system. Its facilities can accommodate most severely disabled children, except for the absolutely worst cases who are in semi-coma or on respirators or for another reason require one-on-one care all the time. For the latter group there are state-run total-care institutions.

One particular morning Adachi arrived at 7:00 A.M., an hour before the children were due, to get paperwork and other chores out of the way. Her first patient was two-year-old Ruby, a hypotonic little girl. The muscles of such children have almost no tone, so they flop around like rag dolls; they cannot sit up by themselves or keep their heads up easily. Unless considerable effort is made to assist them, they simply collapse and just lie there. The doctor had prescribed physical therapy three times a week, but Ruby got it only twice because the center was understaffed.

When she went out to meet the school buses, Adachi found that Ruby, lying in a red wagon, propped against another child, was waiting to be taken to her classroom. Ruby's face had a blurry look; her eyes move but do not see; she is blind, probably deaf, and unresponsive. The hearing aid she wears does not seem to improve her reactions, as far as Adachi can tell, although Ruby's family thinks it helps.

Adachi scooped the plump child out of the wagon with a cheerful greeting and carried her to one of the classrooms, where she put her on a table and changed her diaper. Then she lifted her high, swung her through the air, and sat her down on a mat facing a floor-length mirror. One of her goals was to get Ruby to sit up by herself. The staff hoped that, eventually, Ruby would feed herself, use a potty, and crawl. Those were the goals, but she could not even put her hands down to crawl. Placed in a crawling position, she just flopped over.

Adachi manipulated the child's legs and placed them in a side-sitting position, to encourage more varied use of her muscles. She held her by the waist, let go a little, held her again, and helped her put her arms out for support. She held her securely atop a large green ball and slowly moved it in an atttempt to elicit some balancing responses in her trunk and arms. She bounced her briefly on her lap, then put her down on her hands and knees, encouraging Ruby to hold herself up. Ruby whimpered but her face showed no change of expression.

"Oh, it's hard," Adachi said to her, with acknowledgment but no pity. "But think of the big breakfast you had. We say, please don't feed you all that butter, but they don't know what to do with you so they just give you more." Adachi talks to the children as though they understand because she can't be sure they don't. And she talks as she thinks, so there are no hidden messages. She knows that though they may not comprehend the words, they are highly sensitive to feeling. Ruby stayed on her hands and knees a moment, then flopped to the side.

"I know. The world is such a confusing place. You don't hear much, you don't see, you just tub up," said Adachi. "It will all make a little more sense after a while." Ruby's face was on the mat. Adachi bent her leg, rolled her over from the hip. She was putting Ruby through motions that come naturally and independently to other children, and as she did so she kept talking, calling Ruby by name. Adachi's voice was calm and positive, genuinely cheerful.

231

"Come on, you just have to learn to get your head up," she admonished, placing a stuffed Donald Duck in front of Ruby, who was lying on her stomach and propped on her elbows. Ruby flopped over.

"This kid will sit like the blob of butter she had for breakfast all day," said Adachi. "You put her in a chair, she'll fall asleep. You put her at a table, she'll sleep. She needs stimulation." It seems that in addition to being severely damaged, this child was depressed. Her mother was depressed. Before Ruby started coming to the center, the mother apparently never talked with the child. It simply did not occur to her to do so. But lately, Ruby had been more alert. "What we really need is more support and education for the parents," Adachi said.

Leaving the floppy Ruby to the classroom aide, Adachi moved on to the next classroom and a very spastic five-year-old boy named Kai. "Kai, Kai," she called in a lilting voice that carried reservoirs of confidence and affection. She collected the boy, who was dressed in jeans and a red shirt, from a low bed where he had been lying on his back. His cry of surprise turned into one of delight as she swooped him around the room. His contorted little mouth grinned. She turned him upside down, bounced him, and swung him through the air. He laughed and she laughed with him. She had been working with Kai for nine months. At first he hated physical therapy, but now he clearly enjoyed it.

"When people say, 'Why do you move these kids so vigorously?'" Adachi later explained, "I say, 'What would it feel like to you if you were stuck in a car for twenty-four hours, cramped in a particular position, and you were finally released?' You would want to stretch, run, do something. You would want to feel some movement and circulation. I think a lot of these kids feel that way. They sit or they stand, and when some human being finally comes they love to move. They need to feel air whizzing by them and themselves going up and down and stretching those muscles and feeling a different relationship between their arms, legs, and their trunk. They're kids, after all."

Kai's eyes see but he has no control over their movement and therefore has trouble with tracking and conjugate vision (eyes working in unison). Nobody knows what is happening with him cognitively. He cannot speak and cannot move voluntarily with any precision. His spasticity is severe and he has had seizures. A full-term baby, he was born asphyxiated, with brain edema and nonfunctioning kidneys. With cardiac massage, immediate intubation, and 100 percent oxygen he was resuscitated. After twenty-four days in an intensive care unit, he was discharged from the hospital.

Kai was one of the children who were about to be mainstreamed, that is, enter a regular school classroom with two or three other handicapped children and their own special education aide. Advocates for the handicapped have long sought mainstreaming as a way to break through these children's isolation and make them a part of the world at large. But some educators believe this is not the best approach and that the better strategy is integration, which moves the children to a normal school site, but keeps them together in separate classrooms. The hazard with mainstreaming is that the classroom program is not strictly focused on the handicapped children and their needs cannot always be central, even though they have a teacher of their own. Adachi worried that they might become "bookends," placed in a corner and forgotten by other children or remembered just as curiosities. On the other hand, the great benefit is that the children can be with their chronological peers for their mutual education. Adachi feels that this alone is worth the risk.

"Don't you dare become a bookend, Kai," she said to the boy. She tried to get him to turn his head to look to the right without straightening his right arm, a hard movement for him because he is strongly affected by a primitive reflex that causes him to extend the arm on the side toward which he looks. Then she put him on his abdomen over a bolster and rolled him back and forth, encouraging him to lift his head and put his arms down toward the floor. She held him in different positions and moved him around, talking to him all the time. It seemed to her that he had improved a little. His shirt bore a picture of roller skates and the command, "Rollerskate." Certainly he will never do that.

As Adachi worked with Kai, the other children in the center were otherwise occupied. Johnny, a twelve-year-old, stood in a "standing chimney," which supported him in an upright position. He was hitting the side of his head with his right hand while trying to get his left into his mouth and missing. There was a rough pink spot on both his cheeks from the many misses, and on his head a hairless spot of flaky skin. If the damage he did to himself got worse, someone might immobilize his elbows with a splint. But the staff wouldn't like to do that because they thought

Johnny might be learning and getting a modicum of enjoyment by moving his arms freely. For example, he had also learned to clap his hands; as he saw Adachi with Kai he did it.

Farther away, a girl about Johnny's age was screeching while bobbing back and forth in a chair. Another girl, her hair beautifully braided by her mother, lay in a rocker, staring at the ceiling. A boy with an arm in an elbow splint lay against the wall. He had been hitting and scratching his face violently. His self-destructive behavior was his response to any change in the family routine. His mother was about to remarry and change her job. He had not been getting his accustomed attention.

Andy, who almost drowned at age three, was lying on his side, immobile and seldom responsive, as he had been for the past six years. He was resuscitated too late to avoid permanent brain damage, but his mother continued to believe that God would make him well. It is not uncommon for parents of severely damaged children to seek solace in the hope of miracles. Richard's mother had done this too. "Jesus came to set captives free," she said, "and if you have a child like this you are a captive. We're supposed to put our faith in Him."

Three-year-old Richard is one of three children at the center whose parents successfully sued for malpractice against obstetricians who prescribed labor-inducing drugs and then did not monitor for signs of fetal distress. The child, who is unresponsive, must be fed through a gastrostomy. Nine-year-old Ruth, whose settlement carried the proviso that her parents not disclose the sum—"It was more money than you can imagine, though," says the mother. "Many millions."—stood in front of the piano, scratching at the case with her index finger. She loves to do this. She also loves to play vigorously on the keys, much the way a preschooler would. At home, she had worn out three electric organs.

The settlements do not mean that the families become rich. They pay for the lifetime support of the child. The family still bears the burden of living with a child who might screech all day and bang on a wall or organ and needs to be cared for by special baby-sitters. Richard's parents cannot be away for more than four hours because baby-sitters will not deal with the gastrostomy tube. Ruth's parents, however, were entitled to thirty-six hours of respite care a month. When they were cut back to fourteen, they fought for and retained the full thirty-six. "I'm one of the few parents who did," said Ruth's mother, who uses much of her time to attend meetings of groups trying to improve the lot of the disabled.

Adachi is impressed by the ability of parents to cope, and by the many ways they adapt to meet the challenges of living with a disabled child. She is also aware that disabled children run a higher risk than others of being abused. "It must take an incredible amount of patience and self-control to put up with being on call every day. It's like having an infant all your life," she reflected.

She strapped Kai into a bolster chair that has a tray attached in front. She put a pillow between Kai and the tray to protect his abdomen and strapped his shoulders back so he would not fall forward and hit his head. She put a towel on top of the tray to catch his drool and placed a couple of bright plastic toys before him. She had to move on to Jane, the smallest of the microcephalics, who was developing scoliosis and should ideally have been handled for a half-hour daily instead of twice a week. There were eleven more children to work with. Later, Adachi took a brief lunch break on a sunny bench. After she went home, she would go for a walk, read, or lie down and listen to music.

Adachi came to her work in a unique way. Born in Japan of American parents, she came to the United States to go to secondary school, attended Smith College for two years, then moved on to the California Institute of the Arts to pursue her interests in dance and sociology. Later she became an elementary school teacher and found herself particularly interested in children with learning problems. With her dancer's eye, she observed that many of them had movement abnormalities. This led her to study for her credentials in special education and eventually graduate from the School of Medicine at the University of California in San Francisco with a degree in physical therapy.

She brings a particular vision to her calling. Her cross-cultural experience, her work in dance, her years of teaching, and her mental and physical discipline gained through years of practicing the Chinese martial art of t'ai chi give her a wide perspective on these children.

"Sometimes I feel they're trapped souls, other times I don't know," she said. "I compare them to myself. I like to move and be able to make my own decisions about where I want to be in space, to get out and work and interact with other human beings. And a lot of these kids will never have that option. They are going to be in spaces to which some human being takes them. But maybe they will feel just as free within the parameters of their environment as I do within mine.

"But it seems to me, a lot of the time, that they are condemned to life. Particularly the kids who can't move; they wait for us to move them. They can't speak; they wait for us to guess what they are saying. A lot of them can't eat very well; they have to wait to be fed. They can't bathe themselves. A lot can't go to the bathroom and take care of that themselves; they have to wait for somebody to come and change their diapers. To me that seems like an incredible hardship to the human spirit, to be that dependent on the sensitivity of others.

"Do they have a lot of pain? I don't know. I think so. But if that is how they are born and all they know? Pain has a lot to do with comparison and with awareness of different levels of comfort. I know if I were in their position I would feel pain. But I know adults who consider themselves in pain in states I would not consider at all painful, that would never keep me home from work. Maybe, for these kids, what they feel is normal everyday experience. But often they look uncomfortable to me. They have deformities and gravity then pulls on their heads at funny angles and causes them to work harder. They work harder in a lot of ways that may be considered painful, exhausting. But I really don't know. I wish I could get into the heads of those kids so I could find out, Do you hurt? Part of the reason I'm interested in this work is that if those children are here and we know so little about them, it is our obligation to find out how they can live on the planet with more ease and more pleasure, because they are dependent on us. I don't know if they feel pain, but they are dependent."

Not infrequently, Adachi wonders whether something is missing from the decision-making process that causes these children to be brought into life. She does not blame doctors. "A lot of them are young, and they are not trained to think about this. They look at a child and see this child needs oxygen, needs an IV. They are looking at an organism and trying to keep it alive. Maybe if they had more exposure to what these kids do as they get older, what we have to offer, what's required of them, maybe they would see that some heroic measures are only briefly heroic and may actually open the gate to a lot of suffering. I do think that a lot of people are going by the technological and legal imperative rather than according to an intuitive ethical sense or personal knowledge of what happens to children like these on a day-to-day basis.

So there will be more and more handicapped children. And I wonder, Will we have the resources and the willingness to take care of them?

"I'm sort of an advocate for these kids. I'm interested in the big push that is on to mainstream or integrate them into schools for normal children. If we are going to incorporate medical heroic measures, then we need to take the whole thing.

"If we allow a child to die, in some ways that is a finite decision because we don't have to be concerned with maintaining the quality of life for that child for decades. But if we decide that a child is to live, we have to put our buck on that decision and there has to be support until they do die, even if it's at age ninety. If that is not there, we are condemning them to life. I believe they are really sensitive to their environment and how they are treated. They're living beings!

"The older children get less attention because they don't seem to change much, no matter what we do. But maybe—even if they are not going to move through space differently—maybe we can make their space more interesting so they can enjoy themselves. That's what I want. I would love to see these handicapped children look like they're having fun, to see some glint in their eyes— something.

"Sometimes I think, If our society were educated enough, maybe it would not be so bad to be handicapped. It's a matter of where we draw the line in taking responsibility."

A major concern for Adachi, one she shares with most of the people who work with the severely disabled, is that society is drawing ever further away from taking personal responsibility for the consequences of its technology. The damaged children are invisible to most people. The doctors who save their lives in the nursery are rarely the ones who see them later, and parents are encouraged to farm them out. Public financial support is more easily available for foster care or institutions than for biological parents. It is a rare parent who has the time or financial means to provide lifelong personal care for the child at home.

Adachi's last child that day was the one she believes has the most promise—Susan, who, born with a cord wound twice around her neck and having aspirated meconium, was in an intensive care nursery for two months. Susan clearly understands a great deal and can learn. She is lovable, but she has little ability to communicate, except by uttering a few sounds or by laughing or smiling. Her mouth moves like that of a fish, opening wide and closing. Her arms jerk beyond her control. She cannot stand or crawl but she is trying. She tries very hard. She could turn out to be one of those miracle babies, said Adachi, because she is so responsive. That is, she could do much more than she was doing, and she could communicate, perhaps with the help of a new robotic device, even though her severe spasticity will remain. A major factor in her favor is her family, which shares in her care. Two older siblings do a significant part of the clothing and feeding, and her mother and father are very devoted. Her mother once considered having another child, so that someone likely to outlive the parents could assume responsibility for Susan.

"When I tell that to people," says Adachi, "the usual reaction is, Oh, what a horrible burden to put on a child. And in fact it is. But if you don't do that, you are putting the burden on the generation—the generation of that potential sibling. We seem to be more comfortable putting it on a whole generation than on an individual. But part of that equation is that individuals forget their responsibility. They think the government or someone else should do it, but not with their tax dollars. Never having been exposed to this special population, they would probably be appalled if they were to go to a school or institution for the disabled. But they don't. And they consider it a hardship to grow up with that kind of awareness. My feeling is that face-to-face contact with things we don't want to think about is really crucial to our maturity as people and as a community.

"I ask myself—it's something a lot of therapists think of—if I were in one of those bodies—like the body of that drowning victim—would I want to live? I don't think so. And if it were my child, I don't think I would want heroic measures. Of course, when decisions are made, there is no guarantee. You don't know the future; there is no clear right or wrong. Maybe I'd change my mind. But within the parameters of not knowing we still need to make decisions and take responsibility. Wherever you draw the line, you have to take responsibility. "

At birth, very sick, extremely premature, and severely damaged infants are surrounded by adult attendants—medical professionals, concerned parents, other helpers. As they grow older and it becomes obvious that they will not overcome their disabilities, the crowd around them thins. While they are babies, their parents still hope. They do not look so very different from other babies. At age five to ten, many are still appealing enough to be candidates for March of Dimes posters. They are taken to stimulation programs, day care centers, and special schools where the ratio of adults to children can be as good as six or ten to one, where there is physical therapy and other assistance. They are called developmentally delayed, not disabled. The implication is that they are just late bloomers who will grow at their own pace.

By age twelve, some of the extremely disabled may not even look like children anymore, as their bodies and faces twist into unnatural postures and expressions. More of them live in foster homes or pediatric nursing facilities because their parents have given up the struggle to keep them within the family. A sizable proportion of their families have dissolved under the stress of trying.

At age twenty-two, some of the badly handicapped live in large state hospitals that have been renamed development centers but nevertheless remain what they were: shelters for people of minimal capacity, with no other place to go. Many kind attendants work in such institutions and they are not necessarily worse for their residents than smaller community-based licensed facilities, where most of the seriously disabled are placed, with public aid. Some of the disabled live in board-and-care homes, attend adult programs, or are occupied in sheltered workshops. If they are wheelchair-bound, suffer uncontrolled seizures, or are otherwise too difficult for board and care, they are placed in intermediate or skilled nursing facilities.

By the time these disabled persons are chronological adults, they may be sharing one adult caretaker with six to eighteen others. There is usually no more hands-on attention from physical therapists because no more improvement can be anticipated. The caretakers are expected to perform daily exercises designed to prevent deformities from getting worse, but the caretakers are underpaid and not strictly supervised. Gradually, the totally dependent vanish from society's view. Yet they remain just as needy as they were as children.

Where shall the line be drawn? The question is posed in intensive care nurseries. Is a 20 percent chance of survival enough to begin aggressive life support of a very premature baby, or should the estimate be 50 percent? Is a 70 percent chance of life as a custodial patient enough to cease heroics, or must one be 95 percent sure? Must one go on, anyway, as long as there is any chance for any kind of life, even such as none of the decision makers would accept for themselves? Who shall decide and how?

These questions, so compelling to those with the burden of choice at the threshold of life, do not speak to the larger issue, What of the lives that are saved? The line drawn at birth must be followed beyond the walls of the nursery and beyond the follow-up clinic, into the lives of damaged children as they proceed, day to day, into adulthood. Wherever that line is drawn, it must be followed. The points at which it is drawn are not nearly as important as that it be drawn in relationship to what is to follow.

Whose task is that? Can the neonatologist be expected to do it? His job description does not include it. Can the parent? Certainly not without help from others. The legislator? He needs public pressure. Who shall do it and how shall it be done? Do we agree with the use of medical technology for the purpose of "salvaging" thousands of children who will go on, for many years, fed through naso-gastric tubes and gastrostomies, unable to participate in our communities or meet their own most basic needs, tended at public expense? These questions stand before society because the choice has been made to "save" infants who are born unprepared to survive with ordinary nurture. It is only when these questions are truly addressed that we will become fully responsible in using neonatal care technology to "rescue" infants who are born dying.

CONCLUSION

The truth is that biological science has taken us into a
new world, and it is full of amazements. The risk now is
hubris; we have to guard ourselves henceforth against
overconfidence, and we will have to go carefully before
we begin applying some of the things we are beginning
to learn about.

Lewis Thomas[1]

The purpose of today's training is to defeat yesterday's
understanding.

Miyamoto Musashi[2]
(1584—1645)

The issue in the intensive care nursery is not, as is popularly
perceived, one of deciding who is "worth" saving. Aggressive medical treatment is not a boon that is disbursed to newborns
deemed to deserve it and withheld from others. It is an array of
powerful, violent, dangerous medical technologies available in the
modern hospital. It has been very successful and helped many
infants to survive and grow up healthy; without it, they would
either have died or survived with serious handicaps. It has also
prolonged the dying of others, and sometimes postponed death
indefinitely when life is no longer possible in any meaningful
sense. Intensive care does not, per se, save lives. What it does is
to put infants into a state similar to suspended animation, so
that their physiological processes can be assisted until they recover (in cases of sick babies) or mature (in cases of premature
infants) and may be able to survive on their own. The potential
for recovery or growth must exceed the harm being done by the
artificial life-support system. The harm inflicted by this technology is serious, and it is often difficult for the physician to know
when it has become too great.

Physicians who order intensive care for infants assume responsibility for ascertaining, as best they can, that the powerful sets

of techniques they employ serve the function for which they are intended: to help babies recover and grow into complete human beings. When the probability of such an outcome is low, continuance of intensive care becomes unreasonable.

When physicians make medical decisions, they are never completely sure they are right. They can only act in light of their knowledge, experience, and intuition. But in all medical practice, it is assumed that if they ignore statistical probability without sufficient cause, they are acting against their patients' best interests. There is no reason to make an exception to this general rule in the case of neonatology.

To demand that physicians use intensive care technology beyond the point when it is likely to assist with a patient's problems, as the Baby Doe regulations require, is to demand that they violate their professional commitment to do no harm. To argue that infants must be treated aggressively, no matter how great their disabilities, is to insist that the nursery become a torture chamber and that infants unequipped to live be deprived of their natural right to die.

Perhaps such a demand would not be made had American medicine not in large part abandoned the *primum non nocere* principle in favor of the goal of saving life at all costs. This is not strictly something for which physicians can be blamed. It is the consequence of our society's reluctance to accept death as a part of life, and of a value system that admires and rewards technological innovation far more than the quiet arts of healing. It is also a consequence of economic incentives.

Be that as it may, the standard of care that guides medical practice, and, since 1984, federal law, requires that the physician always choose to err on the side of aggressive treatment with sick and damaged newborns. The results are enormously troubling to many doctors, nurses, and others, most especially parents.

Helen Harrison, author of the excellent *The Premature Baby Book: a Parents' Guide to Coping and Caring in the First Years*, wrote:

> In delivery-room and nursery crises, families have been at the mercy of an accelerating life-support technology and of their physicians' personal philosophies and motives concerning its use. This was my experience seven years ago after the birth of my gravely ill premature son. . . . I have since interviewed numerous parents and physicians who have grappled with similar heartbreaking situations. I sympathize with physicians' concerns when parents re-

quest that there be no heroic measures. However, I sympathize infinitely more with families forced to live with the consequences of decisions made by others. Above all, I sympathize with infants 'saved' for a lifetime of suffering.[3]

The terrible inequities that sometimes occur as a result of intensive care are not likely to be averted as long as policy requires that all newborns be routinely resuscitated in the delivery room and, at the same time, physicians and policymakers remain unwilling to accept death as a merciful outcome. The new technologies have added to the physicians' burden of choice in light of uncertainty. The course of least resistance is to yield to the technological and legal imperatives and uniformly choose to defy the odds by continuing treatment, which is called erring on the side of life. But is it really? A few infants will almost miraculously survive and do well; a far greater number will be condemned to some dim zone of nonbeing. These are infants who, unequipped for a full human life, would have expired without aggressive intervention. The alternative course—the one that under current circumstances requires courage and personal risk—is to allow death when the odds are too grim, accepting the possibility that a rare miracle infant might be lost but knowing that it is far more likely that a child, and its family, are being spared a bleak existence that the doctor would not consider a life. Choosing this course, the doctor knows that, at least, no harm is being done.

It is significant that among the women who work in the Stanford intensive care nursery, several said that if they were to have an extremely premature baby, they would not want it to be treated aggressively. One said that if she knew what was about to happen she would stay away from a hospital with a sophisticated intensive care unit. Others said they would make sure they were under the care of a doctor who would not press to extremes on survival. Many parents would make a similar choice but are not given the opportunity.

Refraining from heroics has been called murder by some who claim to be pro-life. It has been called a violation of God's commandment not to kill. But in effect, the demand that physicians fight death at all costs is a demand that they play God. It is a demand that they try to conquer nature, thereby declaring themselves more powerful than God's order.

The problem is, in part, an obsolete frame of reference. Conquering nature had long been an accepted social goal in Western society. But it fell into disrepute as evidence mounted that nature will have the last word. The popular press and schoolbooks used to be full of praise for Americans who "tamed" rivers by building giant dams, "vanquished" the wilderness, slaughtered Indians. During the rise of industrial society, all nature, including human nature, was viewed as raw material to be brought under control. A popular eighteenth-century writer, James Nelson, advised that "children, while young, may be compared with machines which are or should be set in motion or stopped at the will of others."[4]

Perhaps the ideal of conquest will be replaced by the ideal of living in agreement with nature. The most benign technology works in harmony with natural processes rather than intruding on them. Transistors and solar energy are two examples. Ultrasound and trace gas analysis are others. The obsolete ideal of conquest, however, still hangs on in the concept of war against death, and it is the cause of many of our current ethical problems.

Neonatology is on the frontier of new knowledge, and it demands a new conceptual framework that works in accordance with, rather than against, natural processes. Among other things, it must allow consideration of a fact well known to anyone who has ever grown an apple tree: all fruit that sets cannot ripen. There are always drops. To try to prevent these, or to regret them, would be counterproductive.

In intensive care units, as in new developments in the biomedical sciences, we are seeing more and more that what seemed to be discrete entities are in fact continuing processes. Advancing knowledge and know-how have erased the sharp dividing lines that had seemed to distinguish a fetus from a baby, life from death. Since multiple organ systems can be kept alive now after consciousness appears permanently to have vanished, and since research with other mammals has shown that our species is not exclusively endowed with consciousness, the definition of human life is up for review. The attempt to separate what belongs together leads to distortions in reasoning and practice.

It is as absurd to contend that there is no distinction between a conceptus and a newborn baby as it is to insist that a blastocyst is not life. Both are on the same continuum of human reproduction and of the becoming of a person. It is, for now at least, absurd to argue that a fetus can be protected at the expense of the mother. For until such time as an artificial womb exists, a fetus cannot survive independently of her. A much more difficult question may face us soon: If a defective fetus can be repaired by surgery within the womb, will the mother be required to submit to it?

It is logically inconsistent to argue, as Surgeon General C. Everett Koop did during the Karen Ann Quinlan controversy, that the physician may choose not to start a patient on a respirator, but that once he has started, he may not disconnect it before recovery or brain death without committing homicide.[5] The courts have already vitiated that argument, as has legislation.

Dr. Koop and other advocates of treatment at all costs have based their case on religious and constitutional arguments. The Baby Doe regulations were drawn in light of a particular interpretation of the principle that all men are created equal and are endowed by their Creator with certain inalienable rights, and that among these are life, liberty, and the pursuit of happiness. But is an infant pursuing happiness when, born unequipped for life, he or she is prevented from dying? Would it not be more reasonable to say that life is imposed upon this person? Our forefathers could not have foreseen this situation when they wrote the Declaration of Independence. At that time, they had no need to consider whether there was also a right to die. The issue did not exist, at least in its current form, before the invention of life-support technology.

The civil libertarian stand will not support a full consideration of the dilemmas of intensive care, either with newborns or with older people on the edge of death. It collides with the right to a dignified death which, though not spelled out in the Bill of Rights, is increasingly recognized in law, and with the physician's duty to do no harm. An appropriate frame of reference would include all these, as well as further considerations. For an infant, being unable to speak for herself or himself, is dependent on family and society.

This does not mean that less attention should be given to the protection of the rights of the newborn. Rather, it means that these rights must be considered in their special relationship to the rights of others and in the context in which they are to be exercised. This is true of all rights protected by the Constitution. Supreme Court Justice Andrew Jackson made this point eloquently regarding another constitutional right, that of free speech, in his dissent in the case of *Terminiello v. Chicago*, when he called attention to the fact that the exercise of free speech depends on a community's willingness to accept it and assume whatever burden and risk to public order its protection requires. He concluded, "The preamble declares domestic tranquillity as well as liberty to be an object in founding a Federal Government and I do not think the Forefathers were naive in believing both can be fostered by the law."

For borderline-viable newborns and older persons on the threshold of death, a similar but much more complicated balancing is called for between the constitutionally protected right to life and other rights and responsibilities.

How then do we arrive at the new conceptual frameworks that could help us with the overwhelming dilemmas our success in neonatology has raised? Where no explorer has gone, no map can exist. But it is useful, when old premises are being examined, to look beyond the domain where these premises are found. Medical anthropologist Margaret Lock did this in her study of the ancient tradition of medicine that came from China to Japan and has been thriving alongside cosmopolitan (or Western-style) medical practice. She found it offered insights to Westerners.

Two outstanding features of this medicine, as she describes it in her book *East Asian Medicine in Urban Japan*, are inclusiveness and concern with balance. Neither patients nor their body parts are ever viewed in isolation, as separate entities. They are always considered in relationship to others. Patients are seen as whole persons within their families and "in a continual interchange of energy with the environment," adapting to it rather than trying to overcome it. Patient and family are the principals in the treatment process.

> In the East Asian medical system, the focal point of the healing process is thought of, not as the interaction between doctor and patient, but rather as the sick person at the center of an involved family. Sickness is regarded not as the concern primarily of an individual, but as an event for which the entire family unit has a shared responsibility.[6]

Lock points out that East Asian medicine developed in a cultural milieu different from ours, in a society where people understand themselves in relation to their environment rather than as individuals. Its concepts would not work the same way in another culture. But they invite reflection. Surely stronger links between the nursery and what occurs before, after, and beyond it would prevent some of the problems that trouble us most in neonatology. If we shift our vision so we can observe from a more inclusive perspective, it becomes obvious that integral parts of the picture have been left out.

Why has so little heed been paid to the needs of pregnant women and the babies they carry when the payoff for every dollar invested in prevention of low birth weight is so much higher than that accruing to infants, families, and society from intensive care? There is ample information on how to go about it. If the quotient of imagination and money now invested in efforts to rescue infants after an untimely birth were applied to keeping them inside their mothers for the proper length of time, we would save in manyfold ways. Instead of producing and deploying more neonatologists, this nation needs to send women of sound common sense out into their neighborhoods, to call regularly on women who need support during pregnancy. Some will require only a little friendly advice and encouragement in such efforts as trying to eat properly and resting despite various family pressures, trying to stop smoking or refraining from excessive alcohol consumption. Others will need a ride to the clinic, a respite from their other children for an hour, help with household tasks. Still others will have serious and overwhelming problems with housing, food for the family, unemployment, and other aspects of life, putting the mother-to-be under such great stress that she is at risk of delivering the baby too early. Black women with little formal education and without an adequate income have the highest prematurity rate, so black communities would be the obvious places to begin.

We need to make sure, as much as is possible through public policy, that all women have the opportunity to rest during pregnancy. Toward this end we need a law, such as exists in many other countries, providing time off with pay for women during pregnancy and their child's early infancy, with assurance that they will retain their jobs. We also need adequate information and aid on birth control for teenagers, as was recommended by the Committee to Study the Prevention of Low Birthweight.

Within the medical centers with intensive care nurseries, firm steps should be taken to ensure that parents truly understand their baby's condition, what physicians propose to do, what their choices are, and whether there is any difference of opinion among physicians. This sometimes requires the presence of intermediaries who have the skills and take the time not only to explain but also to listen to parents, comprehend their wishes, and help them be heard by the physicians. In hospitals where the population comes from different ethnic and national backgrounds—which may well include most large urban hospitals in the Western world's large cities—cultural as well as linguistic interpreters should be available.

Within the nursery itself, a more inclusive perspective would reveal that our senses can be dazzled and numbed by technology to such a point as to render us oblivious to basics—such as noise inside the incubator and inside the nursery, and a baby's need for uninterrupted sleep.

For children who emerge damaged from intensive care nurseries, we need to provide such support as will allow development of whatever potential for living and joy they might have, without overburdening their families. It is irresponsible to continue to create a population of handicapped people by medical intervention, with the aid of public funds, without subsequent adequate support for them.

But an inclusive perspective, combined with attention to balance, would also weigh society's commitment to rescuing sick newborns against its commitment to all children. Even as six pediatricians may be standing around one fetus/baby who may or may not grow, 4 million children in the country have no regular source of medical care, 40 percent of all children live below the poverty line, and only one-third of all poor children are covered by Medicaid.

A truly humane society will also heed the fact that while the esoteric art of neonatology is practiced in America, fewer than 10 percent of the children in developing countries are immunized against the six threatening illnesses that immunization can prevent. Five million die annually from lack of immunization, 5 million more of diarrhea. A hundred million daily go hungry.[7]

During the past decades, a quiet movement toward a more inclusive and experience-based way of thinking about social issues has been under way throughout this country. It is one of the most hopeful currents within our society and can be detected in almost any realm one might wish to examine. It is less glaringly visible than the opposite trend toward separation, dispersal, and abandonment of commitment to social justice. The attempt to repair broken connections exerts a mending influence.

In the world of business and finance, a growing number of citizens have begun to assume personal responsibility for the nature of their investments. Until recently, many people who considered themselves socially conscious declined to extend that consciousness to their money's flow. Individuals, labor unions, city governments, and universities looked primarily to the soundest dollar return on retirement funds and other investments, without regard to the work that this money did. Now financial counselors advise people how to earn high interest and simultaneously support such worthwhile projects as high-quality day care for workers' children and environmentally sound development. How strong this trend has grown is evidenced by the move in Congress to require that the United States stop doing business with the Union of South Africa until it abandons its policy of apartheid.

In religion, the Catholic church led in linking religious beliefs and personal behavior when the U.S. bishops issued their statement on nuclear war and followed it with another on the economy. No longer would a parishioner be permitted to give to God on Sunday and work in a defense plant building nuclear weapons during the week without struggling with the contradictions during confession on Saturday. Many other churches assumed personal responsibility for the consequences of U.S. actions abroad by establishing sanctuaries for refugees from Central America, even if that meant trouble with U.S. law.

The movement toward personal responsibility and more inclusive frames of reference has stimulated new thinking about science and medicine. It has brought the patient rights movement, the alternative health movement, and the medical self-care movement. Americans have discovered that (most of the time) they do not really want to think doctors are God—to the relief of many doctors. They have discovered that they must take responsibility for their health.

In the intensive care nursery, the growing understanding that, as John Muir once put it, "everything in the universe is hitched to everything else," demands that the principle *Primum non nocere*, Above all, do no harm, be restored to a position of dominance over the commitment to life saving. If that is done, we will have come a long way.

NOTES

Preface

[1] Donna-Jean B. Walker et al., "Cost-Benefit Analysis of Neonatal Intensive Care for Infants Weighing Less Than 1,000 Grams at Birth," *Pediatrics* 74, 1(July 1984): 20–25.

Chapter One
First Questions

[1] Ernlé W. D. Young, *Societal Provision for Long-Term Needs of the Disabled in Britain and Sweden Relative to Decision-Making in Newborn Intensive Care Units.* (New York: World Rehabilitation Fund, International Exchange of Experts and Information in Rehabilitation, 1984), 20.

Chapter Two
From the Carnival Circuit to High-Tech Circuitry

[1] Leo Stern, "Thermoregulation in the Newborn Infant: Historical, Physiological and Clinical Considerations," in *Historical Review and Recent Advances in Neonatal and Perinatal Medicine*, I, ed. George F. Smith and Dharmapuri Vidyasagar (Mead Johnson Nutritional Division, 1983), 35–36.

[2] Richard D. Wertz and Dorothy Wertz, *Lying-In, A History of Childbirth in America.* (New York: Schocken Books, 1979), 143.

[3] Eugene D. Robin, *Matters of Life & Death: Risks vs. Benefits of Medical Care* (Stanford: Stanford Alumni Association, 1984), 74.

[4] In 1985, after six years spent attempting to gain the approval of the state medical society, Dr. Bell led another move, to mandate that insurance companies pay for preventive health care visits for children through age fifteen. The state legislature subsequently passed such a bill twice, but Governor George Deukmejian vetoed it both times.

[5] Dieter Enzmann et al., "The Natural History of Subependymal Germinal Matrix Hemorrhage," *American Journal of Perinatology* 2, 2 (April 1985): 123–133.

[6] Committee to Study the Prevention of Low Birthweight, Division of Health Promotion and Disease Prevention, Institute of Medicine, *Preventing Low Birthweight.* (Washington, D.C: National Academy Press, 1985), 276.

[7] Charles R. Whitfield, in a talk at the World Symposium of Perinatal Medicine, September 12, 1984, Washington, D.C.

[8] C. Arden Miller, "Infant Mortality in the U.S.," *Scientific American* 253, 1 (July, 1985): 31.

[9] Committee to Study Prevention of Low Birthweight, *Preventing Low Birthweight*, 8.

[10] Penny Glass et al., "Effect of Bright Light in the Hospital Nursery on the Incidence of Retinopathy of Prematurity," *New England Journal of Medicine* 313, 7 (August 15, 1985): 401.

[11] Allen W. Gottfried and Joan E. Hodgman, "How Intensive Is Intensive Care?" *Pediatrics* 74, 2 (August 1984): 292–294.

Chapter Three
The ICN as a Separate Culture

[1] Carol Gilligan, *In a Different Voice: Psychological Theory and Women's Development* (Cambridge: Harvard University Press, 1982), 164–165.

[2] Eugene B. Brody and Howard Klein, "The Intensive Care Nursery as a Small Society. Its Contribution to the Socialization and Learning of the Pediatric Intern," *Paediatrician* 9 (1980): 172.

[3] Ibid., 180.

[4] Coryl LaRue Jones, "Environmental Analysis of Neonatal Intensive Care," *Journal of Nervous and Mental Disease* 170, 3 (March 1982): 140.

[5] Richard E. Marshall, "Complexity: Leadership in an Academic Neonatology Unit," in Richard E. Marshall, Christine Kasman, and Linda S. Cape, *Coping With Caring For Sick Newborns* (Philadelphia: W. B. Saunders, 1982), 83.

Chapter Four
A Miracle Baby

[1] John N. Schullinger et al., "Neonatal Necrotizing Enterocolitis—Survival, Management, and Complications: A 25-year Study," *American Journal of Diseases of Children* 135 (July 1981): 612.

[2] Lucille F. Newman, "Parents' Perceptions of Their Low Birth Weight Infants," *Paediatrician* 9 (1980): 188.

Chapter Six
The Price of Misunderstanding

[1] Alan L. Otten, "Parents and Newborns Win New Legal Rights to Sue for Malpractice," *Wall Street Journal*, June 7, 1985, 1.

Chapter Seven
Death as a Planned Experience

[1] Murray L. Trelease, "Dying Among Alaskan Indians: A Matter of Choice," in Elisabeth Kübler-Ross, *Death: The Final Stage of Growth* (Englewood Cliffs, N.J.: Prentice-Hall, 1975), 36.

[2] Lisa Bain, "Ethics," *USCF Magazine* 72 (June, 1984): 28.

[3] Kübler-Ross, *Death,*, 16.

Chapter Eight
The Limits of Choice

[1] C. Everett Koop, *The Right To Live; The Right to Die* (Wheaton, Ill.: Tyndale House, 1976), 23.

[2] Ibid., 50.

3 Ibid., 79.

4 "America's Abortion Dilemma," *Newsweek*, January 14, 1985, 20–29.

5 Jeff Lyon, *Playing God in the Nursery* (New York: W. W. Norton, 1985), 21–27.

6 Marcia Angell, "Handicapped Children: Baby Doe and Uncle Sam," *New England Journal of Medicine* 309, 11 (September 15, 1983): 660.

7 "Baby Jane Doe at Stony Brook: A Chronology," prepared for a conference, Treatment of Handicapped Newborns: Medical, Ethical, and Social Issues, at State University of New York at Stony Brook, October 17–20, 1984.

8 Ibid.

9 Ibid.

10 Federal Register 49, 238, December 10, 1984, 48163.

11 President's Commission for the Study of Ethical Problems in Medicine and Biomedical and Behavioral Research, "Deciding to Forego Life-Sustaining Treatment: Ethical, Medical, and Legal Issues in Treatment Decisions", (Washington, D.C.: Government Printing Office, March 1983), 217.

12 Ibid., 219.

13 Ibid., 220.

14 Anthony Shaw, "Who Should Die and Who Should Decide?" in *Infanticide and the Value of Life*, ed. M. Kohl (Buffalo, N.Y.: Prometheus Books, 1978), 105–106.

15 Ibid.,

16 Duff, R.S., and A.G.M. Campbell, "Moral and Ethical Dilemmas in the Special-Care Nursery, " *New England Journal of Medicine* 289, 1973: 890–94.

17 John Lorber, "The Doctor's Duty to Patients and Parents in Profoundly Handicapping Conditions," *Medical Wisdom and Ethics in the Treatment of Severely Defective Newborn and Young Children*, David J. Roy, ed., (Montreal: Eden Press, 1978) 16.

18 Ibid.

19 More than three years later, the medical center sent out a press release about a six-month-old boy who had a rare and fatal condition: his intestine could not absorb nutrition from food. "Stanford has solved that problem by intravenous feeding that supplies all the vital nutrients," according to the release. Yet no long-range solution had been found.

20 Benedict M. Ashley and Kevin D. O'Rourke, *Health Care Ethics: A Theological Analysis* (St. Louis: The Catholic Hospital Association, 1978), 242ff.

21 Paul Ramsey, *The Patient as Person* (New Haven: Yale University Press, 1970), xiii.

22 ———. *Ethics at the Edges of Life: Medical and Legal Intersections* (New Haven: Yale University Press, 1978), 219, 225.

23 Joseph Fletcher, "Ethics and Euthanasia," in Robert H. Williams, ed., *To Live and to Die: When, Why, and How* (New York: Springer-Verlag, 1973), 114.

24 Richard A. McCormick, "The Quality of Life, The Sanctity of Life," *The Hastings Center Report* 8, 1 (February 1978), 34–35.

25 Paul Tillich, *Systematic Theology*, vol. 1 (London: Nisbet & Co., Ltd., 1955), 16.

[26] K. Danner Clouser, "The Sanctity of Life: An Analysis of a Concept," *Annals of Internal Medicine* 78, 1 (January 1973): 119ff.

[27] Albert Jonsen, "Do No Harm: Axiom of Medical Ethics," in *Philosophical Medical Ethics: Its Nature and Significance,* ed. S. Spicker and H. T. Englehardt (Dordrecht, Holland: D. Reidel, 1966), 27–41.

[28] McCormick, "Quality of Life," 34.

[29] This right has been recognized by both the American Medical Association and the American Hospital Association. The right to death with dignity was unanimously upheld by a three-judge panel of the California Second Court of Appeals in Los Angeles on December 27, 1984, in the case of William F. Bartling, a seventy-year-old man who was terminally ill and asked that mechanical life support be withdrawn. Glendale Adventist Medical Center, where he was a patient, refused his request, though Mr. Bartling was fully conscious and competent. Mr. Bartling sued the hospital, stating that although he had no wish to die, it was "intolerable" for him to continue to live on the equipment. He demanded to be disconnected from the ventilator "and thereby to permit the natural process of dying to occur—peacefully, appropriately and with dignity." He expired, still on the ventilator, before his case came before the court. But in view of its significance to the nationwide controversy over the right to dignified death, the court heard his posthumous complaint and found in his favor. The decision was relevant to infants as well as to other adults. If Mr. Bartling had lost, guardians of newborns would likely also have lost the right to choose withdrawal of life support when the burden of suffering outweighs hope.

The courts are groping their way through uncharted terrain on this issue. In Ohio, the family of a terminally ill seventy-year-old woman sued a doctor for refusing to disconnect a respirator, arguing that the patient had made known her wish never to be kept alive by artificial means. The doctor insisted that removing life support would be murder. The patient died on the ventilator and the suit was dismissed.

In a 1985 New Jersey case, *In re Claire Conroy*, that state's Supreme Court ruled that life-sustaining treatment may be withheld or withdrawn from an incompetent nursing home patient in the absence of a prior request to die without artificial intervention when the net burdens of the patient's life with the treatment clearly and markedly outweigh the benefits the patient enjoys from life. The procedure requires consent of the patient's guardians, family members, and physicians, as well as state administrative agencies.

Whether intravenous, nasogastric, and gastrostomy feeding are medical procedures or basic forms of care was the issue in a 1983 case before the Superior Court in Orange County, California. The court found that the distinction was based on emotional rather than medical grounds.

[30] Koop, *Right to Live*, 117.

[31] Irving R. Kaufman, "Life-and-Death Decisions," *New York Times*, October 6, 1985, E-21.

Chapter Nine
The Costs and Benefits

[1] Victor R. Fuchs and Leslie Perreault, "The Economics of Reproduction-Related Health Care" (Stanford: 1985: National Bureau of Economic Research, Working Paper No. 1688, manuscript), 11.

[2] C. S. Phibbs et al., "Analysis of Factors Associated with Costs of Neonatal Intensive Care," *Pediatric Research,* 14:438 (1980) (abstract), cited by Peter P. Budetti et al., *The Implications of Cost-Effective Analysis of Medical Technology,* background paper #2: Case Studies of Medical Technologies, #10: "The Costs and Effectiveness of Neonatal Intensive Care" (Washington: Office of Technology Assessment, 1981), 22.

[3] Ernlé W. D. Young, *Societal Provision for the Long- Term Needs of the Disabled in Britain and Sweden Relative to Decision-Making in Newborn Intensive Care Units.* (New York: World Rehabilitation Fund, International Exchange of Experts and Information in Rehabilitation, 1984), 28.

[4] Andrew Wigglesworth, aide to Maryland Governor Harry Hughes, quoted in the *Washington Post,* September 12, 1984, C-1.

[5] Fuchs amd Perreault, "Economics of Reproduction-Related Health Care," 11.

[6] Michael H. Boyle et al., "Economic Evaluation of Neonatal Intensive Care of Very-Low-Birth-Weight Infants," *New England Journal of Medicine* 308, 22 (June 2, 1983): 1130.

[7] Donna-Jean B. Walker et al., "Cost-Benefit Analysis of Neonatal Intensive Care for Infants Weighing Less Than 1,000 Grams at Birth," *Pediatrics* 74, 1 (July 1984): 20–25.

[8] In an account of the brief life and death of their baby, "On the Death of a Baby," *Journal of Medical Ethics* 7 (1981): 5–18, Robert and Peggy Stinson wrote: "He was in effect 'saved' by the respirator to die five long painful, and expensive months later of the respirator's side effects. . . . By the time he was allowed to die, the technology being used to 'salvage' him had produced not so much a human life as a grotesque caricature of a human life, a 'person' with a stunted, deteriorating brain and scarcely an undamaged vital organ in his body, who existed only as an extension of a machine. This is the image left to us for the rest of our lives of our son, Andrew."

[9] Ronald S. Cohen et al., "Favorable Results of Neonatal Intensive Care for Very Low-Birth-Weight Infants," *Pediatrics* 69 (May 1982): 621–625.

[10] ———, "Survival and Morbidity of Our Smallest Babies: Is There a Limit to Neonatal Care?" *Pediatrics* 73, 3 (March 1984): 416.

[11] Toshiko Hirata et al., "Survival and Outcome of Infants 501 to 750 gm: A Six-year Experience," *Journal of Pediatrics* 102, 5(1983): 741.

[12] Marie C. McCormick, "The Contribution of Low Birth Weight to Infant Mortality and Childhood Morbidity," *New England Journal of Medicine* 312, 2 (January 10, 1985): 86.

[13] Sibylle K. Escalona, "Babies at Double Hazard: Early Development of Infants at Biologic and Social Risk," *Pediatrics* 70, 5 (November 1982): 670.

[14] Phyllis S. Glick et al., "Pediatric Nursing Homes, Implications of the Massachusetts Experience for Residential Care of Multiply Handicapped Children," *New England Journal of Medicine* 309, 11 (September 15, 1983): 640.

[15] Ibid.

[16] Paul S. Newacheck et al., "Trends in Childhood Disability," *American Journal of Public Health* 74, 3 (March 1984): 232–236.

[17] Budetti, "Costs and Effectiveness of Neonatal Intensive Care," 19.

[18] Linda Aiken and David Mechanic, eds., "Social Class, Health and Illness," in *Applications of Social Science to Clinical Medicine and Health Policy* (New Brunswick: Rutgers University Press, 1986), 21–22.

Notes

[19] Andrew H. Malcolm, "New Generation of Poor Youths Emerges in U.S.," *New York Times*, October 20, 1985, 1.

[20] Mary O'Neil Mundinger, "Health Service Funding Cuts and the Declining Health of the Poor," *New England Journal of Medicine* 313, 1 (July 4, 1985): 45.

[21] Committee to Study Prevention of Low Birthweight, *Preventing Low Birthweight*. (Washington, D.C.: National Academy Press, 1985), 272.

[22] C. Arden Miller, "Infant Mortality in the U.S.," *Scientific American*, July 1985, 37.

Conclusion

[1] Lewis Thomas, "The Future Place of Science in the Art of Healing," *Journal of Medical Education* 51 (January 1976): 29.

[2] Posted on the wall in Aikido West dojo, Redwood City, California.

[3] Helen Harrison, "Parents and Handicapped Infants," *New England Journal of Medicine* 309, 11 (September 15, 1983): 664–665.

[4] Daniel Beekman, *The Mechanical Baby* (Westport, Conn.: L. Hill, 1977), 60.

[5] C. Everett Koop, *The Right to Live; The Right to Die* (Wheaton, Ill.: Tyndale House, 1976), 105, 107.

[6] Margaret Lock, *East Asian Medicine in Urban Japan* (Berkeley: University of California Press, 1980), 218.

[7] Benjamin José Schmidt, president, International Pediatric Association, São Paulo, Brazil, in a commentary published in *Pediatrics* 74, 2 (August 1984): 294.

SELECTED BIBLIOGRAPHY

Annas, G. "Baby Doe Redux: Doctors as Child Abusers." *Hastings Center Report* 13.5 (October 1983): 26–27.

Beauchamp, T. L., and Childress, J. F. *Principles of Biomedical Ethics,* 2d ed. New York: Oxford University Press, 1983.

Beekman, Daniel. *The Mechanical Baby.* Westport, Conn.: L. Hill, 1977.

Boyle, Michael H., et al. "Economic Evaluation of Neonatal Intensive Care of Very-Low-Birth-Weight Infants." *New England Journal of Medicine* 308, 22 (June 2, 1983): 1330–1337.

Bridge P., and Bridge, M. "The Brief Life and Death of Christopher Bridge." *Hastings Center Report* 11.6 (December 1981): 17–19.

Britton, S. Bennett, et al. "Is Intensive Care Justified for Infants Weighing Less Than 801 gm at birth?" *Journal of Pediatrics* 99, 6 (1981) 937–943.

Brody, Eugene B., and Klein, Howard. "The Intensive Care Nursery as a Small Society. Its Contribution to the Socialization and Learning of the Pediatric Intern." *Paediatrician* 9 (1980): 169–181.

Budetti, Peter P., et al. *The Implications of Cost-Effectiveness Analysis of Medical Technology.* Background Paper #2: Case Studies of Medical Technologies, #10: "The Costs and Effectiveness of Neonatal Intensive Care," Washington, D.C.: Office of Technology Assessment, 1981.

Budetti, Peter, et al. "Trends in Childhood Disability." *American Journal of Public Health* 74, 3 (March 1984): 232–236.

Childress, J. F. *Priorities in Biomedical Ethics.* Philadelphia: Westminster Press, 1982.

Cohen, Ronald S., et al. "Favorable Results of Neonatal Intensive Care for Very-Low-Birth-Weight Infants." *Pediatrics* 69 (1982): 621–625.

Cohen, Sarale E., and Parmelee, Arthur H. "Prediction of Five-Year Stanford-Binet Scores in Preterm Infants." *Child Development* 54 (1983): 1242–1253.

Committee to Study the Prevention of Low Birthweight. Division of Health Promotion and Disease Prevention, Institute of Medicine. *Preventing Low Birthweight.* Washington, D.C.: National Academy Press, 1985.

Comroe, J. H., Jr. "Premature Science and Immature Lungs." In *Retrospectroscope Insights into Medical Discovery.* Menlo Park: Von Gehr Press, 1977, 140–179.

Culver, C. M., and Gert, B. *Philosophy in Medicine.* New York: Oxford University Press, 1982.

Damme, C. "Infanticide: The Worth of an Infant Under the Law." *Medical History* 22 (1978): 1–24.

Darling, R. "Parents, Physicians, and Spina Bifida." *Hastings Center Report* 7, 4 (August 1977): 10–14.

Selected Bibliography

Duff, R. S., and Campbell, A. G. M. "Moral and Ethical Dilemmas in the Special-Care Nursery." *New England Journal of Medicine* 289 (1973): 890–894.

Ellul, Jacques. *The Technological System*. New York: Continuum Publishing Corp., 1980.

Enzmann, Dieter, et al. "The Natural History of Subependymal Germinal Matrix Hemorrhage." *American Journal of Perinatology* 2, 2 (April 1985): 123–133.

Escalona, Sibylle K. "Babies at Double Hazard: Early Development of Infants at Biologic and Social Risk." *Pediatrics* 70, 5 (November 1982): 670–676.

Fletcher, J. *Humanhood: Essays in Biomedical Ethics*. Buffalo: Prometheus Books, 1979.

Fost, N. "Putting Hospitals on Notice." *Hastings Center Report* 12, 4 (August 1982): 5–8.

Gilligan, Carol. *In a Different Voice: Psychological Theory and Women's Development*. Cambridge: Harvard University Press, 1982.

Glass, Penny, et al. "Effect of Bright Light in the Hospital Nursery on the Incidence of Retinopathy of Prematurity." *New England Journal of Medicine* 313, 7 (August 15, 1985): 401

Gorski, Peter A., Davison, Martha F., and Brazelton, T. Berry. "Stages of Behavioral Organization in the High-Risk Neonate: Theoretical and Clinical Considerations." *Seminars in Perinatology* 3, 1 (January 1979): 61–72.

Grobstein, Clifford. *From Chance to Purpose: An Appraisal of External Human Fertilization*. Reading, Mass.: Addison-Wesley, Advanced Book Program, 1981.

Gustafson, J. M. "Mongolism, Parental Desires, and the Right to Life." *Perspectives in Biology and Medicine* 16 (Summer 1973): 529ff.

Harrison, Helen, with Kositsky, Ann. *The Premature Baby Book: A Parents' Guide to Coping and Caring in the First Years*. New York: St. Martin's Press, 1983.

Hirata, Toshiko, et al. "Survival and Outcome of Infants 501 to 750 gm: A Six-year Experience." *Journal of Pediatrics* 102, 5 (May 1983): 741–748.

Horan, D., and Delahoyde, M., eds. *Infanticide and the Handicapped Newborn*. Provo: Brigham Young University Press, 1982.

Jones, Coryl LaRue. "Environmental Analysis of Neonatal Intensive Care." *Journal of Nervous and Mental Disease* 170, 3 (March 1982): 130–142.

Jonsen, Albert R., and Garland, Michael J., eds. *Ethics of Newborn Intensive Care*. A joint publication of Health Policy Program, School of Medicine, University of California, San Francisco, and Institute of Governmental Studies, University of California, Berkeley, 1976.

Jordan, Brigitte. *Birth in Four Cultures*. St. Albans, Vt.: Eden Press Women's Publications, 1978.

Kohl, M., ed. *Infanticide and the Value of Life*. Buffalo: Prometheus Books, 1978.

Koop, C. Everett. *The Right To Live; The Right to Die*. Wheaton, Ill.: Tyndale House, 1976.

Kübler-Ross, Elisabeth. *Death: The Final Stage of Growth*. Englewood Cliffs, N.J.: A Spectrum Book, Prentice-Hall, 1975.

Kulkarni, Prakash, et al. "Postneonatal Infant Mortality in Infants Admitted to a Neonatal Intensive Care Unit." *Pediatrics* 62, 2 (August 1978): 178–183.

Lock, Margaret. *East Asian Medicine in Urban Japan.* Berkeley: University of California Press, 1980.

Lyon, Jeff. *Playing God in the Nursery.* New York: W. W. Norton, 1985.

Marshall, Richard E., Kasman, Christine, and Cape, Linda S. *Coping with Caring for Sick Newborns.* Philadelphia: W. B. Saunders, 1982.

McCormick, Marie C. "The Contribution of Low Birth Weight to Infant Mortality and Childhood Morbidity." *New England Journal of Medicine* 312, 2 January 10, 1985: 82–90.

McCormick, R. "To Save or Let Die: The Dilemma of Modern Medicine." *Journal of the American Medical Association* 229 (1974): 174ff.

Miller, C. Arden. "Infant Mortality in the U.S." *Scientific American* 253, 1 (July 1985): 31–37.

Mohr, James C. *Abortion in America: The Origins and Evolution of National Policy, 1800–1900.* New York: Oxford University Press, 1978.

Murray, T. H. "The Final, Anticlimactic Rule on Baby Doe." *Hastings Center Report* 15, 3 (June 1985): 5–9.

Newacheck, Paul S., et al. "Trends in Childhood Disability." *American Journal of Public Health* 74, 3 (March 1984) 232–236.

Newman, Lucille F. "Parents' Perceptions of Their Low Birth Weight Infants." *Paediatrician* 9 (1980): 182–190.

Newsweek. "America's Abortion Dilemma," January 14, 1985, 20–29.

Poynter, Noel. *Medicine and Man.* Harmondsworth, England: Penguin Books, 1971.

Ramsey, Paul. *Ethics at the Edges of Life: Medical and Legal Intersections.* New Haven: Yale University Press, 1978.

Reich, W., and Ost, D., eds. *Encyclopedia of Bioethics.* New York: Free Press, 1978.

Robertson, J. A. "Involuntary Euthanasia of Defective Newborns: A Legal Analysis." *Stanford Law Review* 27 (1975): 213–269.

———. "Dilemma of Danville." *Hastings Center Report* 11, 5 (October 1981): 5–8.

———. *The Rights of the Critically Ill.* New York: Bantam Books, 1983.

Robin, Eugene D. *Matters of Life & Death: Risks vs. Benefits of Medical Care.* Stanford: Stanford Alumni Association, 1984.

Roy, David J., ed. *Medical Wisdom and Ethics in the Treatment of Severely Defective Newborn and Young Children.* Proceedings of a symposium held on November 18, 1976, organized by the Center for Bioethics, Clinical Research Institute of Montreal, Montreal, Quebec, Canada. Montreal: Eden Press, 1978.

Shaw, M. W., and Doudera, A. E., eds. *Defining Human Life: Medical, Legal, and Ethical Implications.* Ann Arbor: AUPHA Press, 1983.

Silverman, W. "Mismatched Attitudes About Neonatal Death." *Hastings Center Report* 11, 6 (December 1981): 12–16.

———. *Retrolental Fibroplasia: A Modern Parable.* New York: Grune & Stratton, 1980.

Stinson, Robert and Peggy. "On the Death of a Baby." *Journal of Medical Ethics* 7 (1981): 5–18. Later expanded into *The Long Dying of Baby Andrew.* Boston: Atlantic/Little Brown, 1983.

Selected Bibliography

Strong, C. "The Tiniest Newborns."*Hastings Center Report* 13, 1 (February 1983): 14–19.

Swinyward, C. *Decision Making and the Defective Newborn.* Springfield, Ill.: Charles C Thomas, 1978.

Tamub, S. "Withholding Treatment from Defective Newborns." *Law, Medicine, and Health Care* 10 (February 1982): 4–10.

Thomas, Lewis. "The Future Place of Science in the Art of Healing." *Journal of Medical Education* 51 (January 1976): 23–29.

Time. "The New Origins of Life," September 10, 1984, 46–53.

Tooley, M. *Abortion and Infanticide.* Oxford: Oxford University Press, 1983.

Walker, Donna-Jean B., et al. "Cost-Benefit Analysis of Neonatal Intensive Care for Infants Weighing Less Than 1,000 Grams at Birth." *Pediatrics* 74, 1 (July 1984): 20–25.

Weber, L. J. *Who Shall Live? The Dilemma of Severely Handicapped Children and Its Meaning for Other Moral Questions.* New York: Paulist Press, 1976.

Weir, R. *Selective Nontreatment of Handicapped Newborns.* New York: Oxford University Press, 1984.

Wertz, Richard W. and Dorothy C. *Lying-In: A History of Childbirth in America.* New York: Schocken Books, 1979.

Western Journal of Medicine, special issue. "Cross-Cultural Medicine" 139, 6 (December 1983).

Young, Ernlé W. D. *Societal Provision for the Long-Term Needs of the Disabled in Britain and Sweden Relative to Decision-Making in Newborn Intensive Care Units.* New York: World Rehabilitation Fund, International Exchange of Experts and Information in Rehabilitation, 1984.

INDEX

There's an epidemic with 27 million victims. And no visible symptoms.

It's an epidemic of people who can't read.

Believe it or not, 27 million Americans are functionally illiterate, about one adult in five.

The solution to this problem is you... when you join the fight against illiteracy. So call the Coalition for Literacy at toll-free **1-800-228-8813** and volunteer.

**Volunteer
Against Illiteracy.
The only degree you need
is a degree of caring.**

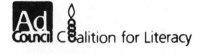 Ad Council Coalition for Literacy